DASH DIET
DETOX

DASH DIET DETOX

14-DAY QUICK-START PLAN
TO LOWER BLOOD PRESSURE AND
LOSE WEIGHT THE HEALTHY WAY

Kate Barrington

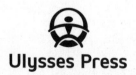

Ulysses Press

Published in the US by:
Ulysses Press
P.O. Box 3440
Berkeley, CA 94703
www.ulyssespress.com

ISBN13: 978-1-61243-521-3
Library of Congress Control Number: 2015944217

Printed in the United States by United Graphics Inc.
10 9 8 7 6 5 4 3 2 1

Acquisitions Editor: Kelly Reed
Managing Editor: Claire Chun
Project Editor: Alice Riegert
Editor: Rebecca Pepper
Proofreader: Lauren Harrison
Index: Sayre Van Young
Cover design: what!design @ whatweb.com
Cover artwork: © Bufo/shutterstock.com
Interior design and layout: Jake Flaherty

Distributed by Publishers Group West

CONTENTS

INTRODUCTION

Do you frequently experience gas, bloating, or indigestion?

Do you suffer from chronic fatigue or muscle aches?

*Do you struggle to maintain a healthy weight,
or are you trying to lose weight?*

*Do you have trouble falling asleep at night
or concentrating during the day?*

If you answered yes to any of these questions, your body could be in a state of toxicity right now and you may not even know it. There are many common toxins to which you are likely exposing yourself each and every day. The food you eat, the air you breathe, and the products you use on a daily basis could be loaded with harmful toxins that your body just doesn't know how to handle. The human body is amazing, and it does have a few natural detoxification systems in place to deal with these daily toxins, but when you expose your body to more toxins than it can handle, the excess may be stored in your cells, causing you to experience the symptoms just described.

There are countless fad diets designed to help you "detoxify" your body, but many of them promise unrealistic results and are not founded on any real scientific principles. The DASH diet, on the other hand, is based on dietary protocols set forth by the National Heart, Lung, and Blood Institute, and it may be just the tool you need to detoxify your body and improve your health. The original DASH diet (short for

Dietary Approaches to Stop Hypertension) was created as a tool to help individuals diagnosed with or at risk for hypertension to lower their blood pressure without medication.[1] Because it is founded on the principles of whole-food nutrition, however, the DASH diet provides a great many other benefits as well, including improved nutrition and detoxification. The DASH diet is the foundation upon which the DASH diet detox program was developed.

The DASH diet detox program is not another complicated fad diet that requires you to count calories or obsess over every little thing you eat. This simple 14-day meal plan requires only that you replace the processed foods in your diet with nutritious whole foods like fresh fruits and vegetables, whole grains, and lean protein. By making a few simple changes to your diet and your lifestyle, you can drastically improve your health, detoxify your body, and even lose weight. In the pages of this book you will find the tools and information you need to start following the DASH diet and, in doing so, completely transform your life. If you are ready to experience the benefits of this amazing program, turn the page and keep reading.

PART I

THE DASH DIET DETOX PROGRAM

CHAPTER 1

DASH DIET BASICS

*"The DASH diet is a lifelong approach to healthy eating
that's designed to help treat or prevent high blood
pressure (hypertension). The DASH diet encourages you
to reduce the sodium in your diet and eat a variety of
foods rich in nutrients that help lower blood pressure,
such as potassium, calcium, and magnesium."*

—DASH Diet: Healthy Eating to Lower Your Blood Pressure, Mayo Clinic[2]

Think back, if you can, to all of the foods you ate within the past
24 hours. Did any of them come from a box or a package? Did you
purchase any from a fast-food restaurant? Did you season your foods
with salt or sweeten them with sugar? If you answered yes to any of
these questions, not only are you are likely to end up with high blood
pressure, but you are also at increased risk for a number of chronic
diseases and conditions, including heart disease, type 2 diabetes,
arthritis, asthma, and more. This group of diseases is often referred to
as "lifestyle diseases" because they result from lifestyle choices such as
diet and lack of exercise rather than genetics or other factors.

Hypertension, or high blood pressure, affects about one in three adults
in America—that's about 65 million people.[3] Hypertension can be
very dangerous because it forces your heart to work harder to pump
blood to your organs and tissues. It also causes the walls of your arter-
ies to harden, which could lead to kidney damage or brain hemor-

rhage. High blood pressure is a serious problem that many Americans overlook. Because it is such a common problem in the United States, the National Heart, Lung, and Blood Institute developed a program to help hypertensive adults lower their blood pressure naturally by making healthy changes to their diet. This program is called Dietary Approaches to Stop Hypertension, or the DASH diet. Unlike many fad diets, the DASH diet is intended to be a lifestyle change—a lifelong commitment to eating wholesome and nutritious foods. By making healthy changes to your diet and limiting your intake of sodium, sugar, and saturated fats, you can significantly lower your blood pressure and reduce your risk for developing serious health problems such as heart disease, stroke, and Alzheimer's. In addition to lowering your blood pressure, the DASH diet can provide a number of other health benefits, including improved nutrition and weight loss.[2] As part of a healthy lifestyle, the DASH diet can also lead to detoxification, which in and of itself provides a great many benefits.

What Is the DASH Diet?

As you have already learned, the DASH diet is an eating plan designed by the National Heart, Lung, and Blood Institute to help hypertensive adults lower their blood pressure naturally, without medication. The DASH diet does not require you to obsessively count calories or severely restrict your diet. It is a healthy eating plan that focuses on whole foods and portion control. The average American diet is saturated with unhealthy processed foods, trans fats, added sugar, and sodium.

The DASH diet is not complicated or difficult to follow; it simply requires you to reduce your daily sodium intake and focus your diet on whole foods. Included in the DASH diet are foods like fresh fruits and vegetables, nuts and seeds, fish and poultry, and low-fat dairy products. Also included in the DASH diet are high-fiber foods like beans and legumes, as well as heart-healthy monounsaturated fats like avocado and extra virgin olive oil.[4] Although this diet plan does not require you to count calories if you do not want to, there are recommendations for the number of servings you should consume from each food group on a daily basis. Tracking your caloric intake will help you to achieve the right balance of these foods and to ensure that your daily nutritional needs are met. You will learn more about the foods included in the DASH diet and the recommended daily servings in the next chapter.

Benefits of the DASH Diet

Although the DASH diet was originally developed to help individuals lower their blood pressure, it provides many additional benefits. The DASH diet was not originally intended for temporary use, as many fad diets are. It was developed as a lifestyle change that can and should be maintained for life. The DASH diet detox is designed to help get you started with the DASH diet so you can enjoy lasting benefits for improved health and wellness. There is both a 14-day and a 28-day plan. The 14-day plan is designed to give you a taste of the DASH diet so you can determine whether or not it is right for you. The longer 28-day plan is designed to give you a firm foundation in starting the DASH diet, helping you to rid your body of toxins so you can receive the maximum benefit from the diet. Simply put, the longer you follow the DASH diet, the more benefits you will receive and the healthier you will become.

Some of the many results you are likely to see when following the DASH diet may include the following:

- Lowered blood pressure—by as much as 12 points within two weeks
- Reduced low-density lipoprotein ("bad" cholesterol) levels
- Improved nutrition resulting from consumption of whole foods
- Reduced intake of sodium and added sugars

- Improved portion control and healthier eating habits
- Reduced risk for chronic diseases like diabetes, heart disease, and stroke
- Healthy weight loss or weight maintenance
- Fewer kidney problems, including kidney stone formation

Many of the benefits associated with the DASH diet result from improved nutrition, portion control, and other healthy eating habits. If you already suffer from high blood pressure—defined as blood pressure higher than 140/90 mmHg—the DASH diet can help you to reduce your blood pressure by as much as 7 to 12 points in as little as two weeks.[3] If you do not currently have high blood pressure, this diet can help you to prevent it. By consuming wholesome, nutritious foods and monitoring your portions, you can boost your nutrition, which will improve your overall health and well-being. Another important benefit of the DASH diet is detoxification. By removing toxin-laden foods such as fast foods, processed foods, and fried foods from your diet, you can detoxify your body. You will learn more about the detoxification benefits of the DASH diet in the next chapter.

The DASH Diet for Weight Loss

In addition to reducing blood pressure levels, many people turn to the DASH diet as a tool for weight loss. Even though the DASH diet was not created for this purpose, following a diet of healthy foods and minding your portions can support weight loss in overweight individuals and healthy weight maintenance in others. How does the DASH diet help you to achieve your weight-loss goals? Because this diet focuses on nutritional foods like fresh fruits and vegetables, lean protein, and low-fat dairy, it is naturally lower in calories than the average American diet. By removing processed and fatty foods from your diet and replacing them with nutritious, low-calorie options, you can decrease your daily caloric intake, which is the key to weight loss.[2] The beauty of the DASH diet is that you do not need to starve yourself to receive these benefits—many of the foods included in the diet are naturally low in calories but high in nutritional value, so you could end up losing weight without even trying.

If you intend to use the DASH diet for weight loss, however, you will achieve better results if you are intentional about the number of calories you consume on a daily basis. Your daily calorie needs will vary depending on your sex, age, and activity level.[5] For example, if you have a job that requires you to be on your feet most of the day, you will naturally burn more calories than a person with a desk job and, as such, your calorie needs will be higher. Men typically have higher calorie needs than women because they have more muscle mass, and muscle burns more calories than fat. In addition, your calorie needs decrease slightly with age as your metabolism slows down. Below you will find a chart detailing the average calorie needs of men and women of different ages and with different activity levels. Keep in mind that these numbers are intended for use as a reference point—your individual calorie needs will vary according to other factors such as weight and body composition.

CALORIC REQUIREMENTS				
Calories Needed to Maintain Current Weight, by Age, Sex, and Activity Level				
	AGE (in years)	SEDENTARY*	MODERATELY ACTIVE**	HIGHLY ACTIVE***
Female	19 to 30	2,000	2,000 to 2,200	2,400
	31 to 50	1,800	2,000	2,200
	Over 51	1,600	1,800	2,000 to 2,200
Male	19 to 30	2,400	2,600 to 2,800	3,000
	31 to 50	2,200	2,400 to 2,600	2,800 to 3,000
	Over 51	2,000	2,200 to 2,400	2,400 to 2,800

* Sedentary refers to individuals who engage only in very light activity, typically as part of their day-to-day routine. An individual with a desk job who does not exercise would be classified as sedentary.

** Moderately active refers to individuals who exercise at a light to moderate level about one to three times per week. Walking at a casual to brisk pace for 20 to 30 minutes counts as moderate activity.

*** Highly active refers to individuals who exercise at a moderate to high level three to five times per week and those who have a job that requires them to spend most of the day on their feet.

The basic equation for weight loss is "calories in < calories out." Essentially, you will lose weight if you consume fewer calories than your body burns on a daily basis. Conversely, if you eat more calories than your body burns, you will gain weight.[5] The chart provides an estimate of the calories the average adult needs to consume to maintain his or her weight. To lose weight, you will need to create a calorie deficit by consuming fewer calories than you need for weight maintenance. It is important, however, not to go below your body's minimum caloric needs, because doing so could result in serious health problems. Your body's minimum calorie requirement is referred to as your basal metabolic rate (BMR)—this is the number of calories your body needs on a daily basis to maintain basic metabolic functions such as respiration and digestion.

Let's step through the process of calculating the number of calories you'll plan to consume daily if you want to lose weight. First, we'll look at how to calculate your BMR. Using that number, you can determine the number of calories you would consume on a daily basis to maintain your current weight. Once you have that number, you can subtract from it to create the calorie deficit necessary to spur weight loss. Keep in mind that 1 pound of fat is equal to about 3,500 calories. So, if you want to lose 1 pound per week, you should subtract about 500 calories from your daily intake. Remember, you can create a calorie deficit not only through reducing your calorie intake, but also through adding exercise to your daily routine. If you have only a few pounds to lose, however, you should limit your calorie deficit to about 300 calories so you do not lose weight too quickly. Numerous studies have shown that the more slowly you lose weight, the more likely you are to keep it off for the long term.

To calculate your BMR, use one of the equations listed below. These calculations are based on the Harris-Benedict formula. This formula was first developed in the early 1900s by James Arthur Harris and Francis Gano Benedict and revised in 1984 to improve its accuracy. It is the formula used most often to calculate BMR and estimated daily calorie requirements using an individual's weight, height, age, and activity level. You will notice that two different equations are listed—one for men and one for women. Men and women require different equations because men typically have a leaner body mass and higher calorie needs than women, and women tend to have higher body fat percentages and lower calorie needs.

Women: BMR = 655

+ (4.35 × weight in pounds)

+ (4.7 × height in inches)

− (4.7 × age in years)

Men: BMR = 66

+ (6.23 × weight in pounds)

+ (12.7 × height in inches)

− (6.8 × age in years)

For example, a 25-year-old woman weighing 135 pounds with a height of 5 feet 4 inches would calculate her BMR as follows:

BMR = 655

+ (4.35 × 135)

+ (4.7 × 64)

− (4.7 × 25)

BMR = 655

+ 587.25

+ 300.8

− 117.5

BMR = 1,425.55 or about 1,425 calories

Once you've calculated your own BMR, you need to factor in your activity level to determine the number of calories you can consume daily to maintain your current weight. Below you will find a list of five different activity levels and the number by which to multiply your BMR for each one:

Sedentary (desk job with little to no exercise)

= BMR × 1.2

Light activity (light exercise 1 to 3 times a week)

= BMR × 1.375

Moderate activity (moderate exercise 3 to 5 times a week)

= BMR × 1.55

High activity (vigorous exercise 6 to 7 times a week)

= BMR × 1.725

Extra activity (physical job + daily exercise or exercise twice daily)

= BMR × 1.9

Using the example of the 25-year-old woman, you would multiply her BMR (1,425) by her activity level. If this woman were sedentary, her daily calorie needs would be about 1,710 calories; if she were moderately active, her daily calorie needs would be about 2,209 calories. After you've calculated your daily calorie needs to maintain your current weight, you can subtract between 200 and 500 calories from that number to determine the number of calories you should consume daily to encourage weight loss. Remember, you should not go below your BMR, so if subtracting 500 calories results in a number that is too low, increase your target calorie intake accordingly.

CHAPTER 2

WHAT IS THE DASH DIET DETOX?

"The DASH eating plan is rich in fruits, vegetables, fat-free or low-fat milk and milk products, whole grains, fish, poultry, beans, seeds, and nuts. It also contains less salt and sodium; sweets, added sugars, and sugar-containing beverages; fats; and red meats than the typical American diet."

—Your Guide to Lowering Your Blood Pressure with DASH, U.S. Dept. of Health and Human Services[3]

When you bite into a juicy hamburger or munch on a handful of chips, you may be aware that these foods are not "good" for your body, but you may not realize just how bad they really are. Processed foods, convenience foods, and fast foods are loaded with artificial ingredients that can fill your body with dangerous toxins. If you take a peek at the ingredients list on the back of the package, you will find things like high-fructose corn syrup, monosodium glutamate (MSG), partially hydrogenated soybean oil, and other unrecognizable ingredients. The fact of the matter is that artificial ingredients like preservatives, sweeteners, dyes, and flavorings often contain dangerous chemicals that can put your body into a state of toxicity.[6]

But what does that toxicity look like? You can't see it when you look in the mirror, and you may think you feel completely fine after eating these foods. If you look a little deeper, however, you may be able to recognize some of the signs of toxicity. Some of the most common signs of toxicity include the following:

- Chronic fatigue
- Joint pain and muscle aches
- Sinus congestion or frequent sinus infections
- Bloating, gas, and constipation
- Diarrhea or foul-smelling stools
- Difficulty falling asleep or staying asleep
- Problems with focus and concentration
- Food cravings
- Water retention, trouble losing weight
- Rashes, psoriasis, or eczema
- Acne and other skin problems
- Dark circles under the eyes
- PMS or other menstrual disorders
- Bad breath (halitosis)

Where Do Toxins Come From?

In an article titled "Toxins and the Immune System," registered nurse Janice Wittenberg defines toxins as "poisonous manmade compounds, or those occurring in nature, or found in the body in the form of microorganisms that have an adverse impact on immune function."[7] Toxins take many forms—you can find them in processed foods, in polluted air, in cleaning products, even in the beauty products you use every day. To understand where toxins come from, start with the different categories into which they can be divided—lifestyle toxins, environmental toxins, and internal toxins.[8] The following sections give examples of toxins belonging to each category. As you review this list, keep a count of how many of these products or substances you encounter on a daily basis.

Lifestyle Toxins

Included in the category of lifestyle toxins are those substances that we willingly put into our bodies. Also included here are factors that can lead to a state of toxicity in the body.[8] Lifestyle toxins include:

- Processed foods, fast food, fried foods
- Prescription drugs and over-the-counter medications
- Processed/enriched grains and refined sugars
- Artificial sweeteners, preservatives, and flavorings
- Antibiotic- and hormone-treated foods
- Genetically modified foods (GMOs)
- Alcohol, caffeine, and other addictive substances
- Nutrient-deficient diet
- Commercially produced beauty products
- Cigarettes and/or cigars
- Engaging in an unhealthy lifestyle, such as lack of exercise or sleep

You may be surprised to learn that your body can become toxic not only as a result of what you ingest, but also as a result of certain lifestyle choices. If you do not get enough sleep or exercise, for example, your body may not function as well as it should, and it could enter a state of toxicity as a result. Without adequate sleep and exercise, you are more likely to experience certain signs of toxicity like digestive issues, chronic fatigue, and skin problems.

Environmental Toxins

It is estimated that about 6,000 new chemicals are added to the Chemical Society's Chemical Abstract list each week. That equates to more than 300,000 new chemicals each and every year. Many of these chemicals can be found in the air we breathe and the water we drink.[14] Environmental toxins include:

- Household cleaning products
- Chemical pesticides and herbicides
- Naturally occurring mold and fungus
- Chemically treated or contaminated water
- Heavy metals and phthalates (found in plastic)
- Air pollution, acid rain, and smog

Internal Toxins

In addition to man-made toxins, there are many toxins that are biologically natural. Toxins with a biological origin are referred to as biotoxins; some examples include neurotoxins and various forms of hemotoxin or necrotoxin found in the venom of snakes, spiders, and scorpions. The human body even produces toxins as a by-product of certain biological processes.[8] Examples of internal toxins include:

- Ammonia and carbon dioxide produced through digestion
- Excess cortisol and negative effects of prolonged stress
- Overgrowth of intestinal flora (small intestinal bacterial overgrowth, or SIBO)
- Suppression of negative emotions

The idea that negative emotions can have a physical impact on your health and well-being may be new to you, but they are a very common contributor to toxicity. Every emotion that you have corresponds to a certain chemical inside the body. Happiness is directly related to the production and release of serotonin, oxytocin, and dopamine—these are the chemicals that make you feel good. Negative emotions are connected to cortisol—the stress hormone. Elevated cortisol levels, especially if they remain elevated over long periods of time, can contribute to a number of health problems, including blood sugar imbalance, weight gain, immune system suppression, and gastrointestinal issues.

Though toxins come from a variety of sources, the majority of the toxins we ingest come from the foods we eat on a daily basis. Every year, the average American consumes about 14 pounds of food additives like artificial flavorings, colorings, preservatives, antimicrobials, and emulsifiers. The same preservatives that food manufacturers use to keep processed foods from spoiling end up destroying some of the nutritional content of the food. These substances have also been linked to health problems like headaches, nausea, and vomiting. Artificial sweeteners may be low in calories, but they too have been connected to health problems like allergies, behavioral problems, and even cancer.[6] The list goes on and on, but the simple fact is that unless you are intentional about avoiding them, toxins make their way into your body through a variety of different means.

What Happens When Our Bodies Become Toxic?

Your body could be in a state of toxicity right now without you knowing it. However, there are a number of signs of toxicity that are easy to identify.[10] Some of the most common problems associated with toxins in the body include the following:

- Chronic fatigue, even after a full night of sleep
- Bad breath, even with proper dental hygiene
- Difficulty losing weight or unexplained weight gain
- Constipation, gas, bloating, and cramping
- Unexplained muscle aches, pains, and tension
- Headaches or sensitivity related to certain smells
- Acne, dry skin, rash, and other skin problems
- Memory loss or difficulty concentrating
- Depression, anxiety, and other mental problems

Because many of these symptoms also correlate to other health problems, the signs of toxicity are easy to overlook. If you are experiencing any of these problems, however, you may want to think about toxicity as a possible cause. The body has a number of natural detoxification processes in place, but it can only do so much. If your ingestion of toxins exceeds your body's ability to get rid of them, your body could quickly become toxic. Luckily, there are a number of ways to counteract toxicity by making healthy changes to your diet and lifestyle.

The Body's Natural Detoxification Ability

Your body has a natural detoxification system in place that helps it filter out some of the toxins you eat, breathe, and drink. For the most part, your liver, kidneys, and immune system combine to remove toxins from your body at about the same rate that you ingest them. If you ingest too many toxins at once, however, they will be stored in your fat cells and will start to accumulate. There are five different organs or systems in your body that help to remove toxins: the liver, lungs, skin, kidneys, and digestive system.[20] Here is a brief overview of how each of these systems detoxifies your body:

Liver: Your liver is the main detoxification organ in your body, and if it doesn't function properly, it can have a negative effect on all of your other organs and systems. Your liver helps detoxify your body by filtering out toxins and excreting them in the form of bile in a two-stage process.

Lungs: The lungs act as a mediator between the air outside your body and the substances that enter the bloodstream. One way in which your lungs help to filter out airborne toxins is by removing them from the body in the form of carbonic gas that can be exhaled. Toxins that make it into the bloodstream are transported into the lungs, where they pass through the alveoli—tiny air sacs that facilitate the exchange of oxygen and carbon dioxide. Those toxins are then expelled from the body in the form of phlegm that can be coughed up.

Skin: Your skin acts as a sort of physical barrier against certain toxins—those found in water are better able to penetrate the skin than toxins found in oils. Water-based products can be absorbed, and the toxins can be excreted in the form of perspiration. Heavy, oily beauty products sit on top of the skin, which interferes with its natural detoxification ability.

Kidneys: Your kidneys act as a sort of filter for toxins, removing them from the bloodstream and excreting them from the body in the form of urine. The kidneys also help to maintain mineral levels in the body, excreting excess minerals to help control the accumulation of dangerous toxins.

Digestive system: The digestive system is responsible for breaking down the food you eat and absorbing the nutrients. It is also the job of your digestive system to remove and eliminate waste products, including toxins. Dietary fiber plays a key role in this process by binding to the toxins so they can be removed.

In order for your body to combat the toxins you ingest on a daily basis, each of these five systems must be working properly. When one system fails to do its job, the rest of them suffer. The key to ensuring that your body's natural detoxification systems work well is to fuel your body with healthy nutrients and to reduce your intake of harmful toxins. That is where the DASH diet comes in. Not only can the DASH diet help you to lower blood pressure and lose weight, but it is a powerful tool for detoxification as well.

The DASH Diet for Detoxification

The definition of *detox*, according to the Cambridge English Dictionary, is "to stop taking unhealthy or harmful foods, drinks, and other substances into your body for a period of time, in order to improve your health." The terms *detox* and *cleanse* have become buzzwords in our society, and many people equate them not only with recovery from drug and alcohol addiction, but with weight loss as well.

JUICE DETOX

Another popular use of the word *detox* is in conjunction with juicing. Countless celebrities and health professionals endorse juice cleanses for weight loss and detoxification. The idea behind this type of detox is that drinking only fresh juices for a period of several days will give your body time to flush out excess toxins. Juice made from fresh fruits and vegetables requires very little digestion because a majority of the fiber has already been removed, making it easy for your body to absorb the readily available nutrients.

The problem with juice cleanses like this is that they are often very low in calories and may not provide the balance of nutrients your body needs to maintain good health. People who engage in juice cleanses often complain of withdrawal symptoms such as headache, fatigue, and irritability—these are the consequences of a low-calorie diet.

The DASH diet is an excellent tool for detoxification because it is based on wholesome, nutritious foods and naturally excludes many of the food sources highest in toxins. The main food groups included in the DASH diet are fresh vegetables, fresh fruits, whole grains, fat-free or low-fat dairy products, lean protein, nuts and seeds, and fats and oils. Fresh fruits and vegetables play a key role not only in the DASH diet but in detoxifying your body. These foods are rich in vitamins and minerals, especially magnesium and potassium, which are particularly helpful in lowering blood pressure. Cruciferous vegetables like broccoli, cabbage, Brussels sprouts, and kale are also rich in calcium d-glucarate, a phytonutrient that supports natural detoxification processes like glucuronidation. During the process of glucuronidation, water-soluble substances bind to dangerous toxins and chemicals so they can be excreted from your body in the form of bile and urine.

Whole grains provide your body with energy in the form of calories as well as dietary fiber. Not only is dietary fiber important for regulating healthy digestion, but it also binds with certain toxins in your gut, helping to remove them from your body in your stools. Eating high-fiber foods will also help you to feel fuller for a longer period of time, which may keep you from snacking during the day and eating extra calories that could lead to weight gain.

Lean protein is another important part of the DASH diet for detoxification. Healthy sources of protein include lean meats, poultry, fish, and seafood. You can also get some protein from low-fat or nonfat dairy products, as well as nuts, seeds, and legumes. Protein plays an important role in supporting your body's detoxification abilities by helping to facilitate cellular growth and repair, counteracting the damaging effects of certain toxins on your cells.

To use the DASH diet for detoxification, you do not necessarily have to follow a strict dietary protocol. The majority of the detoxification benefits you receive from this diet will be a natural result of improved eating habits. When you stop filling your body with processed foods and fried foods, your body will be able to "catch up" in a way. Because you will not be adding to your body's level of toxicity by eating these foods, your organs will be able to process and eliminate the excess toxins that have been stored in your fat cells. Improving your dietary habits will also help to support detoxification by fueling your body with healthy nutrients that will keep your liver, kidneys, and intestines (your body's main detoxification organs) in good shape so they can do the job they were made to do.[17]

You should note that while it is natural to experience some level of withdrawal when you remove certain foods from your diet, if you do a detox right, the benefits will outweigh the consequences. After a few days of following a healthy detox diet, your body will get used to the dietary changes and you will start to feel better.

DASH Diet Detox Rules and Restrictions

Now that you understand how the DASH diet helps to support your body's natural detoxification abilities, you are ready to learn the specifics of the DASH diet detox program. The DASH diet detox is a bit different from the original DASH diet—it has been simplified in terms of the foods you should eat and avoid, as well as the number of servings you should aim for from each food group. There are six steps you need to learn and follow to be successful with the DASH diet detox program.

1. Learn which foods to avoid or eat in moderation. You also need to familiarize yourself with which foods you can eat freely on the diet.

2. Learn the number of servings you should consume from each food group every day based on your daily calorie needs (as calculated in the previous chapter).

3. Start to cook with certain herbs and spices that have natural detoxification benefits. This includes spices like cinnamon, cumin, ginger, and turmeric, as well as herbs like cilantro and peppermint.

4. Begin monitoring your sodium intake according to the recommendations included in the DASH diet.

5. Stay hydrated throughout the entirety of your detox.

6. Incorporate regular exercise into your weekly routine to help maximize your detoxification.

Step One: Learn What Foods You Can and Cannot Eat

The first step in following the DASH diet detox program is to familiarize yourself with the foods that are and are not allowed on the diet. As has already been mentioned, the DASH diet is not a restricted-calorie diet, and you do not need to memorize any confusing rules to follow it. There are, however, certain types of foods that you should avoid when following the DASH diet detox. The goal in avoiding these foods is to reduce your consumption of processed grains, refined sugars, unhealthy fats, and sodium for the purpose of detoxifying your body and improving your overall health. The following chart shows foods to avoid on the DASH diet detox as well as foods to enjoy freely or in moderation.[3]

Note: These lists are not exhaustive; they are simply meant as a guide to show you what kinds of foods to avoid while following the DASH diet detox. You will find a more extensive list of approved foods in the next chapter in the form of a shopping list.

FOOD RULES AND RESTRICTIONS		
EAT FREELY	**EAT IN MODERATION**	**AVOID**
• Fresh fruits, frozen fruits, dried fruits* • Fresh vegetables, frozen vegetables* • Whole grains: Brown rice, whole-grain bread, whole-wheat pasta • Lean meats: Lean cuts of beef, such as sirloin, top round, and bottom round; chicken and turkey; lean fish such as salmon, trout, and cod; shellfish • Low-fat or fat-free dairy products • Dairy-free alternatives • Nuts and seeds • Beans and legumes • Fresh herbs • Dried spices • Fruit juice (unsweetened) • Herbal tea, decaffeinated tea • Water	• Grass-fed butter, trans fat–free margarine • Olive oil, coconut oil, and vegetable oils • Table salt (less than 1 teaspoon per day) • Alcoholic beverages (women no more than one per day, men no more than two) • Caffeinated beverages (no more than two per day) • Natural sweeteners, like coconut sugar, honey, maple syrup, and stevia (no more than 6 tablespoons per week)	• Refined and processed foods: Fast food, baked goods made with all-purpose flour, baking mix, cake flour, or pastry flour; pasta made with enriched flour; sugary breakfast cereals; refined grains (like white rice) • High-fat dairy products: Whole milk, heavy cream, whipped cream, full-fat cheese, butter • Processed and fatty meats: Fatty cuts of red meat (such as filet mignon, porterhouse, and ribeye), lunch meats/deli meats, bacon, smoked meats, and cured foods • Canned foods (except low- or no-sodium items): Soups, vegetables, tomato products, fruit in syrup • Store-bought condiments* • Frozen dinners • High-sodium foods: Pickles, pickled foods, smoked meats, cured foods, sardines, anchovies, olives • Sugar and sweets: Refined sugars, artificial sweeteners, sugary beverages, cakes and pastries, candy

* When it comes to canned goods like fruits and vegetables or store-bought condiments and dressings, you may still be able to use them as long as they are labeled low or no sodium and they do not have added sugar. You should also avoid products made with artificial flavors and dyes when possible.

Step Two: Learn How Many Servings to Have

The second step in following the DASH diet detox is to learn the number of servings you should be consuming on a daily basis from each food group. Again, the DASH diet detox is a bit different from the DASH diet. Rather than trying to reach a certain number of servings per day from each food group, you should strive to meet certain daily recommendations. This will make the detox easier to follow because you will have more freedom in terms of the meals you choose to eat each day. In the DASH diet detox, it is more important to improve your eating habits overall than to meet specific serving recommendations. The goal is to balance your diet with an assortment of fresh fruits and vegetables, whole grains, low-fat dairy, lean protein, nuts/seeds, and healthy fats.[2]

The chart on page 24 details the recommended number of servings for each category per day based on daily calorie intake. The number of servings you eat from each group will vary depending on your daily calorie allotment, so make sure you calculate your daily calorie needs before using the chart.

SERVINGS PER DAY BY FOOD GROUP

FOOD GROUP	1,600 CALORIES	2,000 CALORIES	2,600 CALORIES	SERVING SIZE	EXAMPLES
Fruits	4	4 to 5	5 to 6	1 medium fruit (such as apple, orange, banana) ½ cup fresh fruit ½ cup fruit juice ¼ cup dried fruit	Apples, bananas, grapes, oranges, mangos, melons, peaches, pineapple, berries
Vegetables	3 to 4	4 to 5	5 to 6	1 cup raw leafy greens ½ cup raw vegetables ½ cup cooked vegetables ½ cup vegetable juice	Broccoli, carrots, beans, kale, potatoes, spinach, squash, tomatoes, sweet potato
Whole grains	6	6 to 8	10 to 11	1 slice bread ½ cup cooked rice or cereal	Whole-wheat bread, whole-wheat pasta, oatmeal, brown rice, cereal
Low-fat and fat-free dairy	2 to 3	2 to 3	3	1 ounce cheese 1 cup milk or yogurt	Skim milk, low-fat buttermilk, reduced-fat cheese, low-fat yogurt, fat-free sour cream
Lean meat, poultry, fish	3 to 6	6 or fewer	6	1 egg 3 ounces meat	Flank steak, sirloin, pork tenderloin, chicken, turkey, fish, shellfish
Nuts, seeds, and legumes	3 per week	4 to 5 per week	1	1½ ounces nuts 2 tablespoons nut butter or seeds ½ cup cooked legumes	Almonds, peanuts, walnuts, peanut butter, lentils, black beans, chickpeas
Fats and oils	2	2 to 3	3	1 teaspoon oil 1 tablespoon mayonnaise 2 tablespoons salad dressing ¼ small avocado	Margarine, canola oil, olive oil, coconut oil, low-fat mayonnaise, light salad dressings
Sweets and added sugars (optional)	4 or fewer	6 or fewer	2 or fewer	1 tablespoon jelly or jam 1 tablespoon sugar	Hard candies, maple syrup, white sugar, sorbet

Step Three: Cook with Detoxifying Herbs and Spices

Any dietitian will tell you that the key to following any diet for the long term is to maintain variety—if you get bored, you will be much more likely to stray. Using certain herbs and spices in your DASH diet detox recipes will keep your taste buds happy as well as your body. Fresh or dried herbs and spices are a great way to add flavor to your meals, and they can also provide detoxification benefits to support your DASH diet detox. The following 12 herbs and spices are known for their detoxification benefits.

Cardamom: Cardamom is a spice commonly used in Indian cuisine. It helps to rid your body of harmful bacteria without affecting the beneficial bacteria that regulate digestion in your intestinal tract. Cardamom also has natural mood-boosting benefits.

Cayenne: You probably know of cayenne pepper's ability to spice up a dish, but you may not know about its amazing detoxification and weight-loss benefits. This spice helps to speed your metabolism and aid your digestion—important factors in weight loss as well as detoxification. Adding cayenne to your favorite dishes will help to move things along in your digestive system so toxins are removed quickly without having time to accumulate.

Cilantro: Cilantro is a fresh herb that is also known as coriander leaf. (The seeds of the cilantro plant are the spice known as coriander.) It has a very high antioxidant content and has been shown to help inhibit oxidation in cells. Additionally, cilantro binds to toxic heavy metals like cadmium, mercury, aluminum, and lead to make it easier for your body to get rid of them. Because cilantro is rich in flavor but low in calories, it makes a great addition to the DASH diet detox.

Cinnamon: Most commonly used in baked goods, cinnamon is a spice made from the ground bark of the cinnamon tree. This spice provides the best detoxification benefits when used in conjunction with other healthy ingredients. Detox smoothies and shakes are the best way to incorporate this spice into your DASH diet detox.

Cumin: Cumin is a seed that can be used whole in recipes or ground into powder. This spice supports detoxification by aiding digestion to help flush toxins from the body in your stools. Cumin can also help to boost immune system health, support healthy blood sugar levels, and combat insomnia. This spice is a common ingredient in Indian cuisine and is also widely used in African and Latin American cuisines.

Garlic: Garlic can be used fresh or dried, or can be ground into powder, and it provides a great many benefits. In addition to having natural antioxidant, anti-aging, and anti-inflammatory benefits, garlic is a powerful ingredient for detoxification. It also helps to oxidize toxic heavy metals, making them more water soluble so they can be flushed from the body.

Ginger: Ginger is technically a root that can be used fresh or dried and ground into a powder. One of the main benefits of this spice is that it helps to increase your body's absorption of vitamins and minerals from the food you eat. Detoxification is not just about ridding your body of toxins—it is also about improving the function of your body's organs and systems for maximum health and wellness. By increasing your absorption of essential nutrients, ginger helps to support this goal. Ginger is also a great digestive support, helping to relieve the gas and bloating that some people experience during the early stages of a detox.

Horseradish: The main benefit of horseradish is that it helps to improve your liver function, increasing the liver's ability to filter out carcinogenic substances. In turn, this reduces your risk for developing cancerous tumors and helps to keep existing tumors from growing. Horseradish also helps improve your liver's ability to filter out other dangerous substances.

Peppermint: Peppermint is an herb that can be used fresh or dried. It provides many natural benefits for healthy digestion (an important part of your body's natural detoxification system). Another way to incorporate peppermint into your DASH diet detox is through the use of peppermint essential oil—add it to a detox smoothie or use it with aromatherapy.

Rosemary: In addition to having a pleasing aroma, rosemary tastes great and offers excellent detoxification benefits. This herb can be used fresh or dried, and it works well in combination with other detox herbs and spices. Rosemary contains natural antioxidant properties that help to defend your cells against free radical damage; this not only reduces your risk for cancer and heart disease, but also helps to improve your total body function.

Saffron: Saffron is a spice that is largely used in Eastern cuisine as well as traditional medicine. It has been shown to help reduce blood pressure and to aid digestion—it also supports healthy bladder and kidney function. Both of these organs play an essential role in your body's natural detoxification process, helping to flush toxins from the body in the form of urine.

Turmeric: The main detoxification benefit of turmeric is that it supports healthy liver function. As you have already learned, the liver plays a key role in your body's natural detoxification system. Adding turmeric to your diet will help to boost liver function in addition to providing anticancer and anti-inflammatory benefits. The active ingredient in turmeric is curcumin, a compound that has natural anti-inflammatory, antioxidant, and heart health benefits. Turmeric is the main ingredient in curry powder, and it can be used in a variety of recipes.

Add these herbs and spices to your list of foods to enjoy freely on the DASH diet detox, and use them to flavor your favorite dishes. You will find them used often in the recipes provided later in this book.

Step Four: Limit Sodium

The third step in following the DASH diet detox program is to make an effort to reduce your sodium, or salt, intake. Sodium is an essential nutrient for good health, but consuming too much of it may put you at risk for developing certain health problems. Processed and packaged foods are often very high in sodium, with one serving providing nearly all of (or more than) your daily recommended limit.[12] This is why removing processed foods from your diet is such an important part of the DASH diet detox. Excess sodium in the diet may cause the kidneys to have difficulty filtering excess sodium out of the blood. When this happens, the body begins to retain water to help dilute the sodium and, as fluid levels rise, blood volumes rise as well. The higher your blood volume, the harder your heart has to work and the more pressure is placed on your blood vessels. Over time, the extra pressure may cause your blood vessels to stiffen and, as your heart works harder to pump blood, you could develop high blood pressure and an increased risk for heart attack and stroke.[13]

Before you decide to cut sodium out of your diet, keep in mind that your body does require a certain amount of it. It can be more important to balance your potassium levels with your sodium intake than to decrease your sodium intake. Potassium and sodium have opposite effects on your heart—while increased sodium intake will raise your blood pressure and increase your risk for heart disease, high potassium intake can help decrease blood pressure and relieve some of the pressure in your blood vessels. If you drop your sodium intake too much without also altering your potassium intake, you could end up doing more harm than good.[14]

According to the DASH diet recommendations set forth by the National Heart, Lung, and Blood Institute, you should aim for a daily sodium consumption of around 2,300 milligrams—this is equivalent to about 1 teaspoon of table salt. For individuals with high blood pressure or at risk for high blood pressure, a lower sodium intake of 1,500 milligrams is recommended.[3] You need much more potassium than you do sodium—around 4,700 milligrams per day. This equates to a sodium-to-potassium ratio of about 1:2. If you take a look at the average American diet, however, you will find that most people have a daily sodium-to-potassium ratio closer to 1:0.7, consuming 3,500 milligrams or more of sodium each day but only about 2,600 milligrams of potassium.[14]

Removing processed foods from your diet is the best thing you can do to lower your sodium intake. Processed foods tend to be very low in potassium, so ditching those foods may also help you to improve your sodium-potassium balance. Eating more unprocessed foods like whole grains and fresh produce will help you to get more potassium in your diet in relation to sodium, as long as you avoid overseasoning your foods with table salt. Some of the best natural sources of potassium include broccoli, avocado, asparagus, Brussels sprouts, papaya, bananas, cantaloupe, and pumpkin.[16]

By now you should have a thorough understanding of what the DASH diet is and how you can use it to cleanse your body of harmful toxins. Removing processed foods from your diet is an important part of the first step in following the DASH diet detox program, and it will have the greatest effect in improving your health. In addition to reducing your consumption of processed foods and added sugar, you should pay attention to how many servings you eat each day from the main food categories. The chart provided earlier in this chapter will help you to determine your daily goals. In the next chapter you will receive more practical tips for getting started with the DASH diet detox program. Not only will you receive tips for preparing your DASH diet kitchen, but you will also find detailed shopping lists and tips for eating out while adhering to the detox program restrictions.

Step Five: Stay Hydrated

Another key factor of the DASH diet detox is the focus on hydration. Water is an essential part of any detox because it helps to carry essential nutrients to your cells, aids in healthy digestion, helps to support healthy kidney function, and flushes toxins and wastes out of the body. In addition to these benefits, drinking water keeps your joints properly lubricated and cushioned and helps to regulate your metabolism for steady calorie burn throughout the day.

As you learned earlier, the kidneys play an essential role in your body's natural detoxification system. What you may not know is that water is vital to the process through which your kidneys filter out waste. Each time your heart beats, about 20 percent of the blood it pumps goes to your kidneys. That blood is then filtered through the kidneys, with clean blood moving along through your bloodstream while wastes and toxins are secreted in the form of urine. If your body isn't properly hydrated, your kidneys will not have enough water to produce urine, and all of those toxins and metabolic wastes will continue to build up, causing your body to become toxic.

In addition to supporting detoxification, water is an essential element in healthy weight loss. Not only is water a natural appetite suppressant, but it helps your body to metabolize fat as well. It is the job of your liver to take stored fat deposits and to metabolize them into usable energy. When your body isn't properly hydrated, the kidneys will be unable to do their job and the liver will have to take over some of the extra work. As a result, your liver will focus more on eliminating toxins from the bloodstream than on metabolizing those stored fat deposits. When you drink enough water, both your kidneys and your liver will be able to do their jobs and you will receive the benefit of increased fat burn and weight loss.

Recommendations vary with regard to how much water you should be drinking per day. As a general rule, you should plan to consume half as many ounces of water as you weigh in pounds. For example, a 120-pound woman should consume about 60 fluid ounces of water each day—that is about seven-and-a-half 8-ounce glasses of water. Similarly, a 200-pound man should consume 100 fluid ounces of water daily—that is about twelve-and-a-half 8-ounce glasses. To make sure you reach your daily goals for water consumption, you can try filling a large jug of water in the morning and then drinking it throughout the day—you may even want to draw lines on it with a permanent marker, dividing it up by hours of the day.

Step Six: Incorporate Exercise into Your Routine

Any doctor will tell you that the key to wellness is a healthy diet and exercise. Following the DASH diet detox alone may help to improve your health and lower your blood pressure, but you can supercharge your results simply by adding a little bit of exercise to your weekly routine. Adding exercise to your DASH diet detox program will be especially important if weight loss is one of your goals for switching to the DASH diet. Recall that the formula for weight loss is "calories in < calories out." Essentially, you will lose weight if you burn more calories each day than you take in. You can create a calorie deficit by reducing the number of calories you eat each day and by incorporating some exercise to increase your calorie burn.

Remember, you do not need to starve yourself in order to lose weight—you simply need to follow a healthy eating plan (like the DASH diet detox) and make an effort to get some exercise a few times a week. To give you an idea of how important it is to incorporate exercise into your DASH diet detox, consider the results of a study nicknamed the Encore Study. The full name of this study is "Effects of the DASH Diet Alone and in Combination with Exercise and Weight Loss on Blood Pressure and Cardiovascular Biomarkers in Men and Women with High Blood Pressure" (Blumenthal et al.; see the resources at the end of this book). The results of this study, published in 2010, suggest that combining exercise with the DASH diet can lead not only to weight loss, but also to increased reductions in blood pressure.

This study was conducted on a group of 144 overweight or obese individuals. One third of the study participants were assigned to follow the DASH diet alone. Another third followed the DASH diet plus had three supervised exercise sessions per week. The remaining third was asked to continue their usual diet and exercise habits over the course of the four-month study period. At the end of the study, it was found that the individuals who combined the DASH diet with regular exercise had a significantly lower body weight at the end of the study compared to those who followed the DASH diet alone and those who maintained their current habits. The group that followed the DASH diet alone lost an average of 0.3 kilogram, while the group that incorporated exercise lost an average of 8.7 kilograms and those in the control group gained an average of 0.9 kilogram.[15]

Adding exercise to your weekly routine does not need to be difficult. You do not have to become a marathon runner to receive the benefits of exercise. Incorporating exercise into your weekly routine can be as simple as taking a 20-minute walk three times a week or attending a group fitness class at your local recreation center.[16] The following chart gives exercise recommendations for individuals in different age groups from the U.S. Centers for Disease Control and Prevention (CDC):

CDC EXERCISE RECOMMENDATIONS		
CHILDREN (AGE 6 TO 17)	ADULTS (AGE 18 AND OLDER)	PREGNANT/POSTPARTUM WOMEN
• Minimum of 60 minutes of physical activity every day • Include vigorous aerobic activity at least three times per week • Include muscle-strengthening activities at least three days per week • Include bone-strengthening activities at least three days per week	• Minimum of 2½ hours of moderate-intensity aerobic activity or 1¼ hours of vigorous-intensity aerobic activity each week • Include muscle-strengthening activities at least two days a week	• Minimum of 2½ hours of moderate-intensity aerobic activity each week • Vigorous-intensity activity is okay for women who already do this kind of activity • Muscle-strengthening activities if approved by a healthcare provider

In reviewing the activity recommendations above, you may think that 2½ hours seems like an impossible amount of activity to work into your weekly routine. If you work a full-time job and have to take care of a family, you may feel as though you have limited time to fulfill your obligations, let alone add additional obligations like exercise. The important thing to remember is that you do not have to get all of your exercise in at once—all kinds of exercise count, as long as you achieve a moderate or vigorous level of intensity and maintain it for a minimum of 10 minutes at a time. With this fact in mind, think about all of the opportunities you have each day to work in just 10 to 15 minutes of exercise. Why not take a brisk walk around the block during your lunch break or take your dog for a quick jog after work?

Examples of moderate-intensity exercises include brisk walking, water aerobics, doubles tennis, yoga, golf, ballroom dancing, mowing the lawn, shoveling snow, and bicycling at 5 to 10 miles per hour.

Examples of vigorous-intensity exercises include jogging, walking uphill, fast swimming, aerobics, competitive sports, digging or shoveling heavy snow, and fast bicycling.

Incorporating exercise into your weekly routine does not need to be complicated. For example, a strength-training program option can be attending a group fitness class at your local gym/recreational center or creating your own routine. Some great beginner programs are Stronglifts 5x5, the T Nation 8-week Basic Strength Plan, and Starting Strength (by Mark Rippetoe). You can find information about these basic programs on the Internet for free. A strength-training program does not have to be long and drawn out—it could be as short as 30 minutes if you like.

The following charts contain sample exercise plans to give you an idea of what it might look like to meet the CDC's recommendations for physical exercise in adults aged 18 to 64:

SAMPLE EXERCISE PLAN 1						
2½ hours (150 minutes) of moderate-intensity exercise, with 2 days of strength training						
MONDAY	TUESDAY	WEDNESDAY	THURSDAY	FRIDAY	SATURDAY	SUNDAY
Brisk 40-minute walk	40 minutes swimming	Strength-training program	Brisk 40-minute walk	Strength-training program	30-minute sport or exercise class	Rest day

SAMPLE EXERCISE PLAN 2						
1¼ hours (75 minutes) of vigorous-intensity exercise, with 2 days of strength training						
MONDAY	TUESDAY	WEDNESDAY	THURSDAY	FRIDAY	SATURDAY	SUNDAY
Fast 25-minute jog	Rest day	Strength-training program	Fast 25-minute jog	Rest day	Strength-training program	Fast 25-minute jog

SAMPLE EXERCISE PLAN 3						
Combined moderate- and vigorous-intensity exercise, with 2 days of strength training						
MONDAY	TUESDAY	WEDNESDAY	THURSDAY	FRIDAY	SATURDAY	SUNDAY
Fast 15-minute jog	Brisk 30-minute walk	Strength-training program	Brisk 30-minute walk	Strength-training program	Fast 15-minute jog	Rest day

These charts are intended to serve as a basic outline for the type and amount of physical activity you should get each week. You do not need to limit yourself to walking and jogging—there are many types of physical exercise that can be beneficial for health and weight loss, including endurance activities, strength-training exercises, balance exercises, and flexibility exercises.[17] The following list describes the four main categories of exercise, giving examples of each type that you can use to create your own exercise plan:

Endurance (aerobic activity): This type of activity increases your breathing and your heart rate, making your heart and lungs work harder. As you improve your endurance, you improve your overall physical fitness, and it becomes easier for you to carry out your daily activities.

Examples include brisk walking, jogging, yard work, aerobic dancing, swimming, tennis, basketball, football, golf, and martial arts.

Strength training (muscle-strengthening activity): These exercises work your muscles and help them to become larger and stronger.

Examples include lifting weights, resistance training, and bodyweight exercises.

Balance exercises: These exercises often incorporate lower-body strength and core strength in addition to balance to help prevent falls and improve coordination. You can use balance exercises as part of your strength-training program or practice them in addition to it.

Examples include standing on one foot, walking toe-to-heel, tai chi, yoga, and Pilates.

Flexibility exercises: These exercises help you to stretch out your muscles and to improve flexibility, which gives you more freedom of movement and reduces your chance for injury.

Examples include static stretches, ballistic stretches, and yoga.

Keep in mind that the recommendations for physical activity provided by the CDC are just a guideline—they are designed to give you a minimum to shoot for. If you have the time and the dedication to get 30 minutes of exercise every day instead of just a few times a week, more power to you! You are in control of your progress on the DASH diet detox program, and the harder you work, the better your results will be. Do not think of exercise as a chore or as one more thing you have to check off your daily to-do list. Try to make exercise fun by involving the whole family or by enrolling in group fitness classes at a nearby gym. To help yourself stay motivated, you might even want to start keeping a daily or weekly activity log where you record the type and amount of activity you engage in, so you can keep track of your goals.

CHAPTER 3

GETTING STARTED ON THE DASH DIET DETOX PROGRAM

"The DASH eating plan requires no special foods and has no hard-to-follow recipes. It simply calls for a certain number of daily servings from various food groups."

—Your Guide to Lowering Your Blood Pressure with
DASH, U.S. Dept. of Health and Human Services[3]

Hopefully, by now it is clear to you that the DASH diet is not a complicated plan, nor is it just another fad diet. The DASH diet is a healthy lifestyle choice that can not only reduce your blood pressure and your risk for heart disease, but also help you to lose weight and detoxify your body. In the previous chapters, you learned the basics of the DASH diet as well as the founding principles of the DASH diet detox. Now you will receive some detailed information about getting started with the program, including tips for preparing your DASH diet kitchen, stocking your pantry, and transitioning into a DASH diet eating plan. You will also receive some helpful information about avoiding withdrawal symptoms and for eating out on the DASH diet detox plan. By the time you finish this chapter, you will have a thorough understanding of the DASH diet detox plan and will be ready to get started.

Preparing Your DASH Diet Kitchen

The DASH diet is not intended to be a short-term diet plan or a rapid weight-loss solution—it is designed to be a long-term lifestyle choice that will help you to lower your blood pressure and reduce your risk for heart disease. The DASH diet detox is a simplified version of the DASH diet, and it comes in a 14-day and a 28-day version. If you are not sure whether you want to commit to the DASH diet for the long term, the 14-day detox is a great way to get a taste of the diet without fully committing. If you are serious about making a permanent switch to the DASH diet, the 28-day detox program will get you started on the right foot by detoxifying your body over a period of 28 days.

Because the DASH diet detox plan is intended for long-term use, you should make an effort to start your detox off right, thus maximizing your chances for success. Commit yourself fully to this program by ridding your kitchen and pantry of all the foods that are excluded from the diet. By ridding your kitchen and pantry of processed foods, refined grains, and artificial sweeteners, you will reduce the temptation to stray from the diet by indulging in these foods.

Before cleaning out your kitchen and pantry, review the list of foods excluded from the DASH diet on page 22. You may even want to write it down so you can check each category off the list as you go. Comb your cupboards, pantry, and refrigerator for things like all-purpose flour and baking mixes, high-fat dairy products, high-sodium canned soups and vegetables, frozen dinners and boxed meals, sweetened foods and beverages—anything that doesn't fall into a category of approved foods for the DASH diet detox plan. Once you have gathered up all of these items, get them out of your house. You do not have to throw these items away—donate nonperishable foods to a local food pantry or give them away to family and friends. Do whatever you have to do to rid yourself of these foods so you can start your DASH diet detox program on the right foot.

DASH Diet Shopping List

After you've cleaned out your kitchen and pantry, you will need to restock it with an assortment of DASH diet–approved foods. Take the time to review the general list of approved foods on page 22 and think about which foods you enjoy from each category. The following sample shopping list of DASH diet-approved foods will help you get started.

Fruits and Vegetables

- Fruit, fresh, frozen (unsweetened), dried, or canned in water
- Vegetables, fresh, frozen, dried, or canned in water

Whole Grains

- Amaranth
- Bran cereal
- Brown rice
- Buckwheat
- Bulgur
- Millet
- Muesli
- Oats, old-fashioned or steel-cut
- Quinoa
- Spelt
- Triticale
- Whole-grain or whole-wheat bread
- Whole-grain cereal
- Whole-wheat couscous
- Whole-wheat pasta
- Whole-wheat tortillas
- Wild rice

Meat and Poultry (lean cuts)

- Chicken
- Eggs
- Flank steak
- Ground beef (lean)
- Pork tenderloin
- Sirloin steak
- Turkey

Fish, Seafood, and Meat Substitutes

- Clams
- Cod
- Flounder
- Haddock
- Hake
- Halibut
- Lobster
- Mahi mahi
- Mussels
- Oysters
- Salmon, fresh or canned in water
- Scallops
- Shrimp
- Sole
- Tempeh
- Tofu
- Tilapia
- Tuna, fresh or canned in water
- Whitefish

Dairy (low-fat and fat-free)

- Buttermilk (low-fat)
- Cottage cheese (low-fat)
- Fat-free cheese
- Fat-free cream cheese
- Fat-free evaporated milk
- Fat-free sweetened condensed milk
- Kefir
- Milk (fat-free or low-fat)
- Part-skim mozzarella
- Part-skim ricotta
- Reduced-fat soft cheese, low-sodium (such as Brie, blue cheese, feta, chèvre)
- Reduced-fat hard cheese (such as cheddar, Parmesan, Monterey Jack)
- Sour cream (low-fat)
- Yogurt (nonfat or low-fat)

Nuts, Seeds, and Legumes (raw or dry-roasted, unsalted or lightly salted)

- Almonds, almond butter and flour
- Brazil nuts
- Cashews, cashew butter
- Chestnuts
- Hazelnuts
- Macadamia nuts
- Peanuts, peanut butter
- Pecans
- Pine nuts
- Pistachios
- Soy nuts

- Walnuts
- Chia seeds
- Flaxseed
- Hemp seeds
- Pumpkin seeds
- Sesame seeds
- Sunflower seeds
- Black beans
- Black-eyed peas
- Chickpeas
- Lentils
- Navy beans
- Pinto beans
- Red kidney beans
- Split peas
- White beans

Healthy Fats and Oils

- Avocado
- Mayonnaise (fat-free natural)
- Margarine (trans fat free)
- Almond oil
- Avocado oil
- Canola oil
- Coconut oil
- Flaxseed oil
- Olive oil
- Sesame oil

Detoxifying Herbs and Spices

- Cardamom
- Cayenne
- Cilantro
- Cinnamon
- Cumin
- Garlic
- Ginger
- Horseradish
- Peppermint
- Rosemary
- Saffron
- Turmeric

Pantry and Baking Staples

- Apple cider vinegar
- Balsamic vinegar
- Red wine vinegar
- Rice vinegar
- Rice wine vinegar
- White wine vinegar
- Broths (low sodium)
- Coconut extract
- Coconut, dried (unsweetened)
- Coconut milk, light
- Tomatoes, canned, diced (low sodium)
- Tomato paste (low sodium)

- Tomato sauce (low sodium)
- Applesauce (unsweetened)
- Arrowroot powder
- Baking powder
- Baking soda
- Cocoa powder, unsweetened
- Coconut sugar

- Honey
- Maple syrup
- Stevia
- Vanilla extract
- Whole-wheat baking mix
- Whole-wheat flour

Condiments and Sauces

- Dijon mustard
- Whole-grain mustard
- Fruit spreads (unsweetened)
- Ketchup, organic (low sodium)

- Pesto
- Salad dressing, preservative-free (low sodium)
- Soy sauce (low sodium)

Easing into the DASH Diet Detox

Once you have stocked your pantry and refrigerator with DASH-friendly foods, you can start to ease yourself into the program. If you are the kind of person who usually eats a lot of processed foods, fast foods, and sugary foods, you will want to be very careful about making the transition. Suddenly reducing your intake of high-sugar and high-glycemic foods can result in withdrawal symptoms like headaches, fatigue, and irritability. To avoid these symptoms, you should take a few days, or even a week or more, to transition yourself into the DASH diet detox program. If you usually eat a lot of processed foods and refined carbohydrates, try to slowly reduce your consumption of those foods, replacing them with whole-grain and whole-wheat alternatives. For example, one day you might replace your English muffin with a whole-wheat bagel at breakfast or eat whole-grain granola instead of a sugary breakfast cereal. You can keep the rest of your diet the same for a few days, incorporating this single change, or you can make additional substitutions to further reduce your intake of processed foods.[4] After your body has gotten used to these changes, incorporate the following changes one at a time over the course of several days or weeks, depending how your body reacts:

- Add an extra serving of vegetables to your lunch one day and to your dinner the next day. Maintain the additional servings as you continue to make the transition.
- Replace dessert or an unhealthy snack with a piece of fruit. You can also add a piece of fruit to your breakfast or eat it as a snack.
- Switch over to low-fat or fat-free dairy products. If you are not already eating two to three servings of dairy a day, add one more serving per day until you reach the recommended number of weekly servings.
- Reduce your consumption of red meats by 1 ounce each day until you reach the recommended serving size of 3 ounces per portion.

If you normally eat red meats several times in one week, try cutting back to just one or two portions each week and replace the remaining portions with a leaner source of protein like chicken or fish.

- Start incorporating some meat-free meals into your weekly routine. Begin by replacing one meal per week, working your way up to three to five meat-free meals weekly.
- Focus on whole grains and vegetables as the staples of your meals, with meat almost as a side dish.
- Cut back on table salt when it comes to flavoring your dishes— focus instead on fresh herbs and spices as your main flavoring agents.

Every person's body is different, so you will need to pay close attention to how your body is reacting to the changes you make to your diet. If you choose to incorporate these changes one at a time, it may take you several weeks to fully transition into the DASH diet detox program. If instead you incorporate multiple changes at once, you might make the transition in a matter of days. Pay attention to your body, and do not rush yourself. You will have the rest of your life to follow the program, if you choose. Do what feels right for your body.

TIPS FOR EATING OUT

One of the best things about the DASH diet detox program is that it is not restrictive or complicated to follow. While you should do your best to avoid processed foods and added sugar, there is no rule saying that you can never indulge in a treat once in a while. Many people choose to adhere to the 80/20 rule for dieting—you strive to follow the rules 80 percent of the time but leave yourself a little leeway for mistakes about 20 percent of the time. You should not use this rule as an excuse to "cheat" on the DASH diet, but you should feel free to have the occasional treat or to go out to eat once in a while.[18] If you choose to eat out on the DASH diet, consider these tips:

- Check the menu online ahead of time, if you can, to plan what you are going to order—this will help you to avoid impulsive decisions that might lead you to go off the diet.

- Be on the lookout for ingredients that are likely to be high in fat— this includes fried foods, dishes made with thick or cream-based sauces, meats cooked in butter, and pureed soups.

- Watch out for ingredients that will be high in sodium—this includes dishes prepared with soy sauce, pickled foods, and foods that are smoked or cured.

- Ask that your meal be prepared without salt, and limit your use of high-sodium condiments like table salt, ketchup, mustard, and pickles.

- Go for healthy preparation methods like grilling, broiling, steaming, roasting, or baking—avoid fried foods.

- If bread is served with or before the meal, ask for whole-grain bread and trans fat–free margarine or olive oil instead of butter.

- Choose a healthy side dish like steamed vegetables, fruit salad, or salad with the dressing on the side instead of fries or mashed potatoes.

- If you choose to indulge in dessert, go for a healthier option like fresh fruit, sorbet, or low-fat frozen yogurt—and choose herbal tea or decaffeinated coffee.

The key to success with any diet is to be prepared. If you take the time to remove all items that are excluded from the DASH diet detox program from your kitchen and pantry, you will be less likely to "cheat" while following the program. Stocking your pantry and fridge with healthy, DASH diet–friendly items will ensure that you have healthy ingredients to use in preparing your meals and to enjoy as snacks if you get hungry. Remember, there is no need to rush into the DASH diet detox program. In fact, the more slowly you make your transition, the less likely you will be to experience negative symptoms of withdrawal and the easier you will find it to follow the program for the long term.[2] Making sudden or drastic changes to your diet will undoubtedly have an impact on your body. While you will eventually start to feel healthier and more energetic, you may experience a few bumps along the way. One of the most common side effects of the DASH diet detox is sometimes referred to as the "low-carb flu." As you start to decrease your intake of processed carbs, your body will have to make the switch from burning carbohydrates as fuel to burning fat (particularly stored fat). During this process you may experience withdrawal symptoms such as fatigue, headache, cravings, and irritability. After a few days, however, things should even out and you will begin to feel better. Fat is a more stable source of energy for your body, so once you wean it off of its carbohydrate dependency you will experience fewer energy highs and lows. You will also have fewer cravings for sugar and carbs.

Now that you understand the basics of the DASH diet detox program and the rules for getting started, you are ready to move forward. In the next section you will find a 14-day quick-start guide for the DASH diet detox program. This 14-day program is ideal for people who want to give the DASH diet detox a try without committing to it for a full four weeks (28 days). It will help you to detoxify your body and will get you started on the path toward reduced blood pressure and a healthy heart. If you are serious about maintaining a healthy DASH diet lifestyle, the 28-day DASH diet detox program is the right program for you. This program is inclusive of the 14-day program, with an extra 14 days' worth of meals to ensure that you have a firm foundation in getting started with the DASH diet detox.

CHAPTER 4

THE 14-DAY DASH DIET DETOX PROGRAM

"The DASH diet is flexible and adaptable to your favorite foods, tastes, and lifestyle. DASH is recommended by the 2010 Dietary Guidelines for Americans and ChooseMyPlate.gov as one of the best plans people of all ages can follow to be healthy."

—DASH Diet Eating Plan, www.DashDietOregon.org

While the DASH diet is intended to be used as a long-term lifestyle change rather than a temporary diet, there is no reason why you should rush into it. The DASH diet detox program is designed to ease you into the DASH diet, helping you to improve your eating habits and to flush excess toxins from your body in the process. After reading the previous chapter, you should understand the importance of preparing not only your kitchen and pantry for the switch, but your body as well. If you already follow a healthy diet, transitioning into the DASH diet detox plan may be easier for you than for individuals who subsist on a diet consisting mainly of fast food, processed foods, and other unhealthy food choices. No matter what your current dietary habits are, the DASH diet detox is the perfect way to reboot your eating habits and boost your nutrition, all while reducing blood pressure and cleansing your body of harmful toxins.

If you would like to give the DASH diet detox a try but are not ready to commit to the full 28-day program, this 14-day program may be just what you need. In this chapter you will find a DASH diet detox meal plan that incorporates delicious breakfasts, lunches, dinners, and snacks/desserts for a full 14 days. To follow the 14-day DASH diet detox plan, simply use the shopping lists provided to stock your kitchen and pantry, and then follow the chart, preparing the designated meals each day. Many of the meals and snacks included in this meal plan come from the recipes provided later in this book, but others are just simple meals and snacks that you can prepare on your own or purchase at the store. Feel free to replace these simple meals and snacks with recipes from the book if you have time to prepare an extra meal. If you struggle to find time to cook every day, however, you should also consider spending some time on the weekends preparing your lunches and snacks for the week so you do not have to make them every morning before work. Many of the recipes in this book—particularly soups and salads—can be prepared ahead of time and reheated as needed.

At the end of the meal plan, you will find a tally of the number of servings from each food group for each week. If you need more servings from a particular group (based on your calorie needs calculated in Chapter 1), add a healthy snack or two that fulfills those nutritional requirements. You will find a list of healthy DASH diet–friendly snacks at the back of the book in the Appendix. In addition, the Appendix provides a collection of DASH diet detox smoothies. While following this 14-day plan you should also make sure to drink plenty of water—refer to the weekly serving recommendations chart from Chapter 2 to determine how much water you should be drinking each day.

This meal plan is based on the recommended weekly servings for a 2,000-calorie daily diet. Feel free to adjust it based on your own recommended daily calorie intake.

14-DAY DASH DIET DETOX MEAL PLAN

	BREAKFAST	LUNCH	DINNER	SNACK/DESSERT
WEEK 1				
SATURDAY	Cinnamon Applesauce Baked Oatmeal (page 79) 1 cup fat-free yogurt 1 ounce chopped nuts Whole-wheat English muffin, plain	Apple Almond Chicken Salad (page 133) 2 slices whole-wheat bread 1 cup baby carrots 1 medium orange	Rosemary Roasted Chicken with Vegetables (page 140) Warm Veggie Quinoa Salad (page 167) 1 cup fresh fruit	1 slice Whole-Wheat Banana Chocolate Chip Bread (page 184) 1 medium apple
SUNDAY	Broccoli Cheese Egg Muffin (page 81) 2 slices whole-wheat toast, plain	Open-Faced Tuna Melt (page 109) 2 cups salad greens 2 tablespoons fat-free salad dressing	Baked Eggplant Parmesan (page 136) Leftover Veggie Quinoa Salad Lemon Parmesan Broccoli (page 172)	Merry Peach Mango Smoothie (page 216) 1 cup baby carrots
MONDAY	Whole-wheat English muffin 1 tablespoon trans fat–free margarine 1 cup fat-free yogurt	3 ounces leftover Rosemary Roasted Chicken 2 cups salad greens 2 tablespoons fat-free salad dressing 1 medium apple	Whole-Wheat Lemon Artichoke Pasta (page 147) Garlic Sautéed Spinach (page 175) 1 cup fresh fruit	1 cup fat-free yogurt 1 cup fresh berries 1 ounce almonds
TUESDAY	Leftover Cinnamon Applesauce Baked Oatmeal 2 scrambled eggs 2 slices whole-wheat toast, plain	Roasted Root Vegetable and Cauliflower Soup (page 108) 2 cups salad greens 2 tablespoons fat-free salad dressing	3 ounces grilled chicken breast Mushroom and Kale Buckwheat Salad (page 166) 1 medium apple	Cooling Cucumber Melon Smoothie (page 212) 2 brown rice cakes
WEDNESDAY	1 cup fat-free yogurt 1 cup fresh berries 2 slices whole-wheat toast, plain	3 ounces low-sodium turkey breast on whole-wheat bread 1 cup celery sticks 1 medium orange	Whole-Wheat Margherita Pizza (page 148) Red Cabbage Carrot Slaw (page 169) 1 cup fresh fruit	1 cup fat-free yogurt 1 cup fresh fruit 1 ounce chopped nuts

14-DAY DASH DIET DETOX MEAL PLAN

	BREAKFAST	LUNCH	DINNER	SNACK/DESSERT
THURSDAY	Leftover Broccoli Cheese Egg Muffin Whole-wheat English muffin, plain	Easy Fennel Apple Soup (page 128) 1 cup baby carrots 1 medium banana	3-ounce grilled fish fillet Cilantro Brown Rice (page 170) 1 medium orange	1 slice leftover Whole-Wheat Banana Chocolate Chip Bread 1 medium apple
FRIDAY	1 cup steel-cut oats 1 cup fresh berries 2 slices whole-wheat toast, plain	2 tablespoons peanut butter on 2 slices whole-wheat bread 1 cup baby carrots 1 medium apple	Blue Cheese Turkey Burger (page 141) Leftover Cilantro Brown Rice 1 cup fresh fruit	Berry, Beet, and Apple Smoothie (page 210) 2 brown rice cakes
			WEEK 2	
SATURDAY	Cranberry Almond Breakfast Quinoa (page 87) 2 slices whole-wheat toast, plain 1 cup fresh fruit	Baked Root Vegetable Cakes (page 110) 1 cup baby carrots 1 medium apple	Greek-Style Stuffed Bell Peppers (page 137) Ginger Snap Peas (page 164) 1 medium pear	Blueberry Almond Crumble (page 194) 8 whole-wheat crackers
SUNDAY	Baked Eggs in a Basket (page 94) Whole-wheat English muffin, plain 1 cup orange juice	Cranberry Feta Chicken Sandwich (page 107) 1 cup celery sticks 1 cup fresh fruit	Ginger Shrimp and Vegetable Stir-Fry (page 146) 1 cup Cilantro Brown Rice (page 170)	Cinnamon Baked Apple Chips (page 189) 1 cup baby carrots
MONDAY	1 cup whole-grain breakfast cereal 1 cup fat-free milk 1 medium apple	3 ounces low-sodium sliced ham on whole-wheat pita 1 tablespoon reduced-fat mayonnaise 1 sliced green bell pepper 1 medium apple	3 ounces grilled chicken breast 1 cup Garlic Herb Millet (page 168) 1 medium apple	1 cup fat-free yogurt 1 cup fresh berries 2 brown rice cakes

14-DAY DASH DIET DETOX MEAL PLAN

	BREAKFAST	LUNCH	DINNER	SNACK/DESSERT
TUESDAY	Roasted Red Pepper and Feta Omelet (page 93) Whole-wheat English muffin 1 tablespoon fat-free margarine 1 medium banana	Pear and Butternut Squash Soup (page 124) 1 cup fat-free yogurt 1 cup fresh fruit	Whole-Wheat Penne with Fresh Pesto (page 149) Sesame Sautéed Kale (page 170) Cucumber Red Onion Salad (page 172)	1 Cherry Date Energy Ball (page 188) 8 whole-wheat crackers
WEDNESDAY	Cherry Cinnamon Overnight Oats (page 100) 1 medium banana	3 ounces grilled chicken with 3 cups salad greens 2 tablespoons fat-free salad dressing 1 medium apple	3-ounce grilled fish fillet 1 cup leftover Cilantro Brown Rice 1 cup fresh fruit	Cucumber, Kale, and Banana Smoothie (page 214) 2 brown rice cakes
THURSDAY	Whole-wheat English muffin 1 tablespoon trans fat–free margarine 1 cup fat-free yogurt	Southwestern Three-Bean Salad (page 117) 3 cups salad greens 2 tablespoons fat-free salad dressing 1 cup fresh fruit	Grilled Salmon with Mango Cilantro Puree (page 139) 1 cup leftover Garlic Herb Millet	Marvelous Mango Ginger Smoothie (page 219) 2 brown rice cakes
FRIDAY	2 scrambled eggs 2 slices whole-wheat toast, plain	3 ounces tuna on 2 slices whole-wheat bread 1 cup baby carrots 1 medium banana	Tempeh Tikka Masala (page 162) 1 cup leftover Cilantro Brown Rice	1 medium apple 8 whole-wheat crackers

14-DAY DASH DIET DETOX PLAN — WEEKLY SERVINGS				
	DAILY GOAL	WEEKLY GOAL	WEEK 1 TOTAL	WEEK 2 TOTAL
FRUITS	4 to 5	28 to 35	34	33
VEGETABLES	4 to 5	28 to 35	36	34
GRAINS	6 to 8	42 to 48	43	43
DAIRY	2 to 3	14 to 21	16	16
PROTEIN	6 or fewer	18 or fewer	15	15
NUTS/SEEDS	4 to 5 (weekly)	4 to 5	5	5
FATS	2 to 3	14 to 21	15	13
SWEETS	Up to 6 (weekly)	Up to 6	6	6
WATER	16	16 daily	16 daily	16 daily

Week 1 Shopping List (Days 1 to 7)

Fruits and Vegetables

- Apples, Granny Smith—7 medium, 3 large
- Bananas—1 small, 4 medium
- Basil—1 bunch
- Beet—1 small
- Bell pepper, red—1 medium
- Berries, fresh—3 cups
- Blueberries, frozen—1½ cups
- Broccoli, chopped—13 cups
- Cabbage, red—1 medium head
- Carrots, baby—4 cups
- Carrots, chopped—1 cup
- Carrots, shredded—4 cups
- Cauliflower—1 medium head
- Celery—1 bunch
- Chives—1 bunch

- ❑ Cilantro—1 bunch
- ❑ Cucumber, English—1 small
- ❑ Eggplant—1 large
- ❑ Fennel—1 large bulb
- ❑ Fruit, fresh, chopped—5 cups
- ❑ Garlic—1 head
- ❑ Ginger—1 knot
- ❑ Honeydew melon, chopped—1 cup
- ❑ Kale, chopped—5 cups
- ❑ Lemons—2
- ❑ Limes—2
- ❑ Mango, chopped—1 cup
- ❑ Onions, red—2 small
- ❑ Onions, sweet—1 small, 1 large
- ❑ Onions, yellow—3 medium, 1 large
- ❑ Oranges—4 medium
- ❑ Parsley—1 bunch
- ❑ Parsnip—1 medium
- ❑ Peaches, sliced—1 cup
- ❑ Peppermint—1 bunch
- ❑ Rosemary—1 bunch
- ❑ Salad greens, premixed—6 cups
- ❑ Spinach, baby—2 pounds
- ❑ Sweet potato—1 large
- ❑ Tarragon, fresh—1 bunch
- ❑ Tomatoes—2 medium
- ❑ Tomatoes, cherry—1 cup
- ❑ Turnip—1 medium
- ❑ Zucchini—1 small

Poultry, Meat, and Seafood

- ❑ Chicken breast, boneless skinless—12 ounces
- ❑ Chicken breast, grilled—3 ounces
- ❑ Chicken drumsticks and thighs—4 pounds
- ❑ Fish fillet, grilled—3 ounces
- ❑ Tuna, canned in water (low-sodium)—2 (6-ounce) cans
- ❑ Turkey breast, sliced (low-sodium)—3 ounces
- ❑ Turkey, ground, lean—1¼ pounds

Eggs and Dairy Products

- ❑ Cheese, part-skim mozzarella, fresh—1 pound
- ❑ Cheese, part-skim mozzarella, shredded—1½ cups

- ☐ Cheese, reduced-fat blue, crumbled—¼ cup
- ☐ Cheese, reduced-fat cheddar, shredded—½ cup
- ☐ Cheese, reduced-fat cheddar, sliced—4 slices
- ☐ Cheese, reduced-fat Parmesan, shaved—¼ cup
- ☐ Cheese, reduced-fat Parmesan, grated—½ cup
- ☐ Eggs, large—13
- ☐ Egg whites—1 large plus 1 cup
- ☐ Margarine, trans fat–free—3 tablespoons
- ☐ Mayonnaise, reduced-fat—¼ cup
- ☐ Milk, fat-free—1¾ cups
- ☐ Yogurt, fat-free—7½ cups

Grains and Baked Goods

- ☐ Buckwheat, uncooked—¾ cup
- ☐ Buns, whole-wheat, burger—6
- ☐ Bread, whole-wheat—18 slices
- ☐ Breadcrumbs, whole-wheat—2 cups
- ☐ English muffins, whole-wheat—3
- ☐ Flour, whole-wheat, pastry—4 ¾ cups
- ☐ Oats, uncooked, old-fashioned—2 cups
- ☐ Oats, uncooked, steel-cut—1 cup
- ☐ Pasta, whole-wheat, bowtie—12 ounces
- ☐ Quinoa, uncooked—1 cup
- ☐ Rice, uncooked, brown—1 cup
- ☐ Rice cakes, brown—4

Dried, Canned, and Jarred Goods

- ☐ Almonds, sliced—3 tablespoons plus 1 ounce
- ☐ Apple juice, unsweetened—2 cups
- ☐ Applesauce, unsweetened—1 cup
- ☐ Artichoke hearts—1 (14-ounce) can
- ☐ Broth, chicken (low-sodium)—2⅓ cups
- ☐ Broth, vegetable (low-sodium)—8 cups
- ☐ Chocolate chips, reduced-fat—½ cup
- ☐ Seeds, chia—1 tablespoon

- ❏ Seeds, sunflower, toasted—¼ cup
- ❏ Tomato sauce, low-sodium, low-sugar—1 (24-ounce) jar
- ❏ Walnuts, chopped—2 ounces
- ❏ Yeast, active dry—1 packet

Spices, Sauces, and Pantry Items

- ❏ Baking powder
- ❏ Baking soda
- ❏ Black pepper
- ❏ Dried bay leaf
- ❏ Dried Italian seasoning
- ❏ Dried oregano
- ❏ Dried thyme
- ❏ Ground cinnamon
- ❏ Ground cumin
- ❏ Ground ginger
- ❏ Ground saffron
- ❏ Ground turmeric
- ❏ Honey
- ❏ Mustard, Dijon
- ❏ Mustard, whole-grain
- ❏ Oil, coconut
- ❏ Oil, olive
- ❏ Oil, vegetable
- ❏ Peanut butter
- ❏ Salad dressing, fat-free
- ❏ Salt
- ❏ Sugar, coconut
- ❏ Vanilla extract
- ❏ Vinegar, rice

Week 2 Shopping List (Days 8 to 14)

Fruits and Vegetables

- ❏ Apples—6 medium, 4 large
- ❏ Bananas—1 small, 3 medium
- ❏ Basil, fresh—2 cups
- ❏ Bell peppers, green—2 small, 1 medium
- ❏ Bell peppers, red—6 medium
- ❏ Berries, fresh—1 cup
- ❏ Blueberries, fresh—3 cups
- ❏ Broccoli, chopped—1½ cups
- ❏ Carrots, baby—3 cups
- ❏ Cauliflower, chopped—1½ cups
- ❏ Celery—1 bunch
- ❏ Chile, mild green—1 medium

- ❏ Chives, fresh—1 bunch
- ❏ Cilantro, fresh—2 bunches
- ❏ Corn, frozen—1 cup
- ❏ Cranberries, frozen—12 ounces
- ❏ Cucumbers, English—1 small, 4 medium
- ❏ Fruit, fresh, chopped—5 cups
- ❏ Garlic—1 head
- ❏ Ginger—1 knot
- ❏ Horseradish, fresh—1 knot
- ❏ Kale—2 bunches plus 1 cup
- ❏ Lemon—1
- ❏ Limes—5
- ❏ Mangos—2 medium plus 1 cup
- ❏ Mint—1 bunch
- ❏ Mushrooms, sliced—1½ cups
- ❏ Onions, green—7 large
- ❏ Onions, red—3 medium
- ❏ Onions, yellow—3 small, 1 medium, 3 large
- ❏ Parsley—1 bunch
- ❏ Pears—3 medium
- ❏ Peas, sugar snap—1 pound
- ❏ Rosemary—1 bunch
- ❏ Salad greens, premixed—6 cups
- ❏ Shallots—3 small
- ❏ Spinach, frozen—1 (10-ounce) package
- ❏ Squash, butternut—2 pounds
- ❏ Tomatoes, Roma—2 large
- ❏ Zucchini—1 small

Poultry, Meat, and Seafood

- ❏ Bacon, turkey, uncooked—2 slices
- ❏ Chicken breast, boneless skinless—1
- ❏ Chicken breast, grilled—3 ounces
- ❏ Ham, sliced (low-sodium)—3 ounces
- ❏ Salmon, boneless—1½ pounds
- ❏ Shrimp, large uncooked, peeled and deveined—1½ pounds
- ❏ Tempeh, chopped—1 cup
- ❏ Tuna, canned in water (low-sodium)—3 ounces

Eggs and Dairy Products

- ❏ Cheese, reduced-fat cheddar, shredded—⅓ cup
- ❏ Cheese, reduced-fat feta, crumbled—8 ounces plus ¾ cup

- ❑ Eggs, large—8
- ❑ Margarine, trans fat–free—3 tablespoons

- ❑ Mayonnaise, reduced-fat—1 tablespoon
- ❑ Milk, fat-free—6¾ cups
- ❑ Yogurt, fat-free—4½ cups

Grains and Baked Goods

- ❑ Bread, whole-wheat—18 slices
- ❑ Cereal, whole-grain, cold—1 cup
- ❑ Crackers, whole-wheat—24
- ❑ English muffins, whole-wheat—3
- ❑ Flour, whole-wheat, pastry—2 tablespoons
- ❑ Millet, uncooked—¾ cup

- ❑ Oats, old-fashioned, uncooked —½ cup
- ❑ Oats, steel-cut, uncooked—1 cup
- ❑ Pasta, penne, whole-wheat—12 ounces
- ❑ Pita, whole-wheat—1
- ❑ Quinoa, uncooked—1½ cups
- ❑ Rice, brown, uncooked—1 cup
- ❑ Rice cakes, brown—6

Dried, Canned, and Jarred Goods

- ❑ Almonds, slivered—½ cup
- ❑ Beans, black—1 (15-ounce) can
- ❑ Beans, red kidney—1 (15-ounce) can
- ❑ Bell pepper, red, roasted—¼ cup
- ❑ Broth, chicken (low-sodium)—2 cups
- ❑ Cashews, raw—2 cups
- ❑ Cherries, dried, chopped—1½ cups
- ❑ Chickpeas—1 (15-ounce) can

- ❑ Coconut milk, canned, light—1 cup
- ❑ Coconut, unsweetened, shredded—1 cup
- ❑ Cranberries, dried, unsweetened—⅓ cup
- ❑ Dates, pitted Medjool—1 cup
- ❑ Juice, orange, fresh—2 ¼ cups
- ❑ Olives, Kalamata, sliced—¼ cup
- ❑ Pine nuts, raw—⅓ cup
- ❑ Salsa, tomato—1 cup

- ❑ Seeds, sesame, toasted—2 tablespoons
- ❑ Tahini—¼ cup
- ❑ Tomatoes, fresh, diced—1 cup
- ❑ Tomatoes, stewed—2 (14.5-ounce) cans

Spices, Sauces, and Pantry Items

- ❑ Arrowroot powder
- ❑ Black pepper
- ❑ Cayenne
- ❑ Chili powder
- ❑ Dried coriander
- ❑ Dried oregano
- ❑ Garam masala
- ❑ Ground cardamom
- ❑ Ground cinnamon
- ❑ Ground cumin
- ❑ Ground fenugreek
- ❑ Ground ginger
- ❑ Ground saffron
- ❑ Ground turmeric
- ❑ Honey
- ❑ Oil, canola
- ❑ Oil, coconut
- ❑ Oil, olive
- ❑ Oil, sesame
- ❑ Paprika
- ❑ Salad dressing, fat-free
- ❑ Salt
- ❑ Soy sauce, low-sodium
- ❑ Sugar, coconut
- ❑ Vanilla extract
- ❑ Vinegar, rice
- ❑ Vinegar, rice wine

CHAPTER 5

THE 28-DAY DASH DIET DETOX PROGRAM

"It's hard to change a long-standing habit, and a detox program—no matter how long—is one way to put a wedge between your old ways and your new ones. . . . Often if you just try to quit eating [problem] foods you'll have limited success and go back to your old ways. But if you cleanse the body and replace those foods with healthier choices, you can retrain yourself and be more likely to stick to your new habits."

—12 Benefits of Detoxing the Body, Bembu.com[3]

If you are dedicated to cleansing your body of harmful toxins, and you do not have a problem making a long-term commitment, the 28-day DASH diet detox program might be the right choice for you. This program starts with the same 14-day meal plan as the shorter DASH diet detox but includes an extra 14 days' worth of recipes to make sure that you really start your DASH diet detox on the right foot. The 28-day DASH diet detox is ideal for people who want to commit to the DASH diet lifestyle in order to enjoy long-term benefits like reduced blood pressure and improved overall health and wellness. To follow the 28-day DASH diet detox, simply use the shopping lists in this chapter to stock your kitchen and pantry each week and then prepare the designated meals listed for each day. While it may be challenging at first to get used to a new diet, having the pressure of choosing what meals to eat taken off your shoulders can make a big difference in ensuring that you stick to the diet.

This meal plan is based on the recommended weekly servings for a 2,000-calorie daily diet. Feel free to adjust it based on your own recommended daily calorie intake.

28-DAY DASH DIET DETOX MEAL PLAN			
BREAKFAST	LUNCH	DINNER	SNACK/DESSERT
WEEK 1			
SATURDAY Cinnamon Applesauce Baked Oatmeal (page 79) 1 cup fat-free yogurt 1 ounce chopped nuts Whole-wheat English muffin, plain	Apple Almond Chicken Salad (page 133) 2 slices whole-wheat bread 1 cup baby carrots 1 medium orange	Rosemary Roasted Chicken with Vegetables (page 140) Warm Veggie Quinoa Salad (page 167) 1 cup fresh fruit	1 slice Whole-Wheat Banana Chocolate Chip Bread (page 184) 1 medium apple
SUNDAY Broccoli Cheese Egg Muffin (page 81) 2 slices whole-wheat toast, plain	Open-Faced Tuna Melt (page 109) 2 cups salad greens 2 tablespoons fat-free salad dressing	Baked Eggplant Parmesan (page 136) Leftover Veggie Quinoa Salad Lemon Parmesan Broccoli (page 172)	Merry Peach Mango Smoothie (page 216) 1 cup baby carrots
MONDAY Whole-wheat English muffin 1 tablespoon trans fat–free margarine 1 cup fat-free yogurt	3 ounces leftover Rosemary Roasted Chicken 2 cups salad greens 2 tablespoons fat-free salad dressing 1 medium apple	Whole-Wheat Lemon Artichoke Pasta (page 147) Garlic Sautéed Spinach (page 175) 1 cup fresh fruit	1 cup fat-free yogurt 1 cup fresh berries 1 ounce almonds
TUESDAY Leftover Cinnamon Applesauce Baked Oatmeal 2 scrambled eggs 2 slices whole-wheat toast, plain	Roasted Root Vegetable and Cauliflower Soup (page 108) 2 cups salad greens 2 tablespoons fat-free salad dressing	3 ounces grilled chicken breast Mushroom and Kale Buckwheat Salad (page 166) 1 medium apple	Cooling Cucumber Melon Smoothie (page 212) 2 brown rice cakes

28-DAY DASH DIET DETOX MEAL PLAN

	BREAKFAST	LUNCH	DINNER	SNACK/DESSERT
WEDNESDAY	1 cup fat-free yogurt 1 cup fresh berries 2 slices whole-wheat toast, plain	3 ounces low-sodium turkey breast on whole-wheat bread 1 cup celery sticks 1 medium orange	Whole-Wheat Margherita Pizza (page 148) Red Cabbage Carrot Slaw (page 169) 1 cup fresh fruit	1 cup fat-free yogurt 1 cup fresh fruit 1 ounce chopped nuts
THURSDAY	Leftover Broccoli Cheese Egg Muffin Whole-wheat English muffin, plain	Easy Fennel Apple Soup (page 128) 1 cup baby carrots 1 medium banana	3-ounce grilled fish fillet Cilantro Brown Rice (page 170) 1 medium orange	1 slice leftover Whole-Wheat Banana Chocolate Chip Bread 1 medium apple
FRIDAY	1 cup steel-cut oats 1 cup fresh berries 2 slices whole-wheat toast, plain	2 tablespoons peanut butter on 2 slices whole-wheat bread 1 cup baby carrots 1 medium apple	Blue Cheese Turkey Burger (page 141) Leftover Cilantro Brown Rice 1 cup fresh fruit	Berry, Beet, and Apple Smoothie (page 210) 2 brown rice cakes
WEEK 2				
SATURDAY	Cranberry Almond Breakfast Quinoa (page 87) 2 slices whole-wheat toast, plain 1 cup fresh fruit	Baked Root Vegetable Cakes (page 110) 1 cup baby carrots 1 medium apple	Greek-Style Stuffed Bell Peppers (page 137) Ginger Snap Peas (page 164) 1 medium pear	Blueberry Almond Crumble (page 194) 8 whole-wheat crackers
SUNDAY	Baked Eggs in a Basket (page 94) Whole-wheat English muffin, plain 1 cup orange juice	Cranberry Feta Chicken Sandwich (page 107) 1 cup celery sticks 1 cup fresh fruit	Ginger Shrimp and Vegetable Stir-Fry (page 146) 1 cup Cilantro Brown Rice (page 170)	Cinnamon Baked Apple Chips (page 189) 1 cup baby carrots
MONDAY	1 cup whole-grain breakfast cereal 1 cup fat-free milk 1 medium apple	3 ounces low-sodium sliced ham on whole-wheat pita 1 tablespoon reduced-fat mayonnaise 1 sliced green bell pepper 1 medium apple	3 ounces grilled chicken breast 1 cup Garlic Herb Millet (page 168) 1 medium apple	1 cup fat-free yogurt 1 cup fresh berries 2 brown rice cakes

28-DAY DASH DIET DETOX MEAL PLAN

	BREAKFAST	LUNCH	DINNER	SNACK/DESSERT
TUESDAY	Roasted Red Pepper and Feta Omelet (page 93) Whole-wheat English muffin 1 tablespoon fat-free margarine 1 medium banana	Pear and Butternut Squash Soup (page 124) 1 cup fat-free yogurt 1 cup fresh fruit	Whole-Wheat Penne with Fresh Pesto (page 149) Sesame Sautéed Kale (page 170) Cucumber Red Onion Salad (page 172)	1 Cherry Date Energy Ball (page 188) 8 whole-wheat crackers
WEDNESDAY	Cherry Cinnamon Overnight Oats (page 100) 1 medium banana	3 ounces grilled chicken with 3 cups salad greens 2 tablespoons fat-free salad dressing 1 medium apple	3-ounce grilled fish fillet 1 cup leftover Cilantro Brown Rice 1 cup fresh fruit	Cucumber, Kale, and Banana Smoothie (page 214) 2 brown rice cakes
THURSDAY	Whole-wheat English muffin 1 tablespoon trans fat–free margarine 1 cup fat-free yogurt	Southwestern Three-Bean Salad (page 117) 3 cups salad greens 2 tablespoons fat-free salad dressing 1 cup fresh fruit	Grilled Salmon with Mango Cilantro Puree (page 139) 1 cup leftover Garlic Herb Millet	Marvelous Mango Ginger Smoothie (page 219) 2 brown rice cakes
FRIDAY	2 scrambled eggs 2 slices whole-wheat toast, plain	3 ounces tuna on 2 slices whole-wheat bread 1 cup baby carrots 1 medium banana	Tempeh Tikka Masala (page 162) 1 cup leftover Cilantro Brown Rice	1 medium apple 8 whole-wheat crackers
		WEEK 3		
SATURDAY	Egg Baked in Avocado (page 78) 2 slices whole-wheat toast, plain 1 medium banana	Roasted Acorn Squash Soup with Toasted Pecans (page 114) 1 cup baby carrots 1 cup fresh fruit	Cajun-Style Seared Scallops (page 171) Garlic Herb Millet (page 168) Ginger Snap Peas (page 164)	Spiced Carrot Cake Muffin (page 185) 1 medium apple
SUNDAY	Spinach and Red Pepper Frittata (page 83) 2 slices whole-wheat toast, plain 1 cup fresh fruit	Couscous-Stuffed Baked Tomato (page 119) 2 cups salad greens 2 tablespoons fat-free salad dressing	Coconut-Crusted Baked Tilapia Fillets (page 143) Garlic Mashed Cauliflower (page 174) Parmesan Wild Rice Pilaf (176)	Vanilla Almond Rice Pudding (page 191) 2 brown rice cakes

28-DAY DASH DIET DETOX MEAL PLAN

	BREAKFAST	LUNCH	DINNER	SNACK/DESSERT
MONDAY	Whole-wheat English muffin, plain 1 cup fat-free yogurt 1 ounce chopped nuts	3 ounces grilled chicken with 2 cups salad greens 2 tablespoons fat-free salad dressing 1 medium orange	3 ounces grilled chicken breast Amaranth Tabbouleh Salad (page 174) 1 medium apple	Triple Berry Supreme Smoothie (page 211) 8 whole-wheat crackers
TUESDAY	Banana Flaxseed Muffin (page 85) 2 scrambled eggs	Spinach Mozzarella Panini (page 120) 1½ cups celery sticks 1 cup fresh fruit	2 cups fresh spinach 1 cup leftover Parmesan Wild Rice Pilaf 1 cup fresh fruit	Whole-Grain Blueberry Almond Muesli (page 188)
WEDNESDAY	2 slices whole-wheat toast 1 tablespoon trans fat–free margarine 1 cup fat-free yogurt	2 tablespoons peanut butter 1 tablespoon jam 2 slices whole-wheat bread 1 cup baby carrots 1 medium banana	Chicken with Pasta Puttanesca (page 142) Sesame Sautéed Kale (page 170) 1 cup fresh fruit	Cucumber, Kale, and Banana Smoothie (page 214) 2 brown rice cakes
THURSDAY	1 cup fat-free yogurt 1 cup fresh berries 2 slices whole-wheat toast, plain	Chicken, Avocado, Mango, and Quinoa Salad (page 126) 1 cup baby carrots 1 cup fat-free yogurt 1 cup fresh berries	3-ounce grilled fish fillet 1 cup leftover Garlic Herb Millet 1 cup fresh fruit	1 cup fat-free yogurt 1 cup fresh berries 2 brown rice cakes
FRIDAY	Peachy Pear and Pineapple Smoothie (page 222) Whole-wheat English muffin, plain	3 ounces low-sodium sliced turkey breast on whole-wheat pita 1 cup celery sticks 1 medium apple	Chipotle-Lime Grilled Shrimp Skewers (page 153) 1 cup Cilantro Brown Rice (page 170) 1 cup fresh berries	Beautiful Broccoli Kale Smoothie (page 215) 8 whole-wheat crackers
WEEK 4				
SATURDAY	Sautéed Sweet Potato Mushroom Hash (page 86) 1 cup fresh fruit 1 slice whole-wheat toast, plain	Creamy Waldorf Salad (page 124) 1 cup sliced bell pepper 1 medium apple	Black Bean Quinoa Burger (page 152) 2 cups baby spinach 2 tablespoons fat-free salad dressing 1 cup fresh fruit	Orange Pomegranate Brown Rice Pudding (187) 2 brown rice cakes

28-DAY DASH DIET DETOX MEAL PLAN

	BREAKFAST	LUNCH	DINNER	SNACK/DESSERT
SUNDAY	Choco-Coconut French Toast (page 91) 1 cup fresh fruit 1 cup fat-free milk	Tomato, Mozzarella, and Pesto Panini (page 125) 1 cup fat-free yogurt 1 cup fresh berries 1 cup baby carrots	Dijon-Crusted Pork Chop (page 157) Avocado Brown Rice Salad, no peanuts (page 165) 1 medium apple	Maple Raisin Oatmeal Bake (page 190) 1 cup fat-free milk
MONDAY	1 cup steel-cut oats 1 cup fresh berries 1 cup fat-free yogurt	3 ounces low-sodium sliced turkey breast on whole-wheat bread 1 cup celery sticks 1 medium orange	Sweet Potato Veggie Burger (page 144) Grilled Zucchini Slices (page 169) 1 cup fresh fruit	Carrot, Apple, and Ginger Smoothie, no honey (page 211) 2 brown rice cakes
TUESDAY	Tomato Basil Egg White Omelet (page 104) 2 slices whole-wheat toast, plain 1 cup fat-free yogurt	Grilled Portobello Mushroom Burger (129) 2 cups salad greens 2 tablespoons fat-free dressing 1 medium banana	3 ounces grilled chicken 1 cup Cilantro Brown Rice (page 170) 1 cup fresh fruit	1 slice Whole-Wheat Chocolate Zucchini Bread (page 192) 1 cup fat-free milk
WEDNESDAY	1 cup cold whole-grain breakfast cereal 1 cup fat-free milk 1 medium apple	2 tablespoons peanut butter on 2 slices whole-wheat bread 1 cup baby carrots 1 cup fresh fruit	Whole Lemon and Herb Roasted Chicken (page 156) Garlic Sautéed Spinach (page 175) Lemon Parmesan Broccoli (page 172)	Celery, Cucumber, and Lime Smoothie (page 216) 8 whole-wheat crackers
THURSDAY	Leftover Choco-Coconut French Toast 2 scrambled eggs	Sweet Potato and Carrot Soup with Ginger (page 132) 1 cup fresh fruit	3-ounce grilled fish fillet 1 cup leftover Cilantro Brown Rice 1 medium apple	Chili Baked Sweet Potato Fries (page 181) 2 brown rice cakes
FRIDAY	Whole-wheat English muffin 1 tablespoon trans fat–free margarine 1 cup fat-free yogurt 1 cup fresh berries	3 ounces leftover Lemon and Herb Roasted Chicken 2 cups salad greens 2 tablespoons fat-free salad dressing 1 medium apple	3 ounces tuna on 2 cups baby spinach 1 cup fresh fruit 2 brown rice cakes	Pumpkin Pie Smoothie, no honey (page 220) 2 brown rice cakes

28-DAY DASH DIET DETOX PLAN—WEEKLY SERVINGS						
	DAILY GOAL	WEEKLY GOAL	WEEK 1 TOTAL	WEEK 2 TOTAL	WEEK 3 TOTAL	WEEK 4 TOTAL
FRUITS	4 to 5	28 to 35	34	33	35	33
VEGETABLES	4 to 5	28 to 35	36	34	33	36
GRAINS	6 to 8	42 to 48	43	43	43	43
DAIRY	2 to 3	14 to 21	16	16	16	13
PROTEIN	6 or fewer	18 or fewer	15	15	15	15
NUTS/SEEDS	4 to 5 (weekly)	4 to 5	5	5	4	4
FATS	2 to 3	14 to 21	15	13	18	18
SWEETS	Up to 6 (weekly)	Up to 6	6	6	6	6
WATER	16	16 daily	16 daily	16 daily	16 daily	16 daily

Week 1 Shopping List (Days 1 to 7)

Fruits and Vegetables

- ❏ Apples, Granny Smith—7 medium, 3 large
- ❏ Bananas—1 small, 4 medium
- ❏ Basil—1 bunch
- ❏ Beet—1 small
- ❏ Bell pepper, red—1 medium
- ❏ Berries, fresh—3 cups
- ❏ Blueberries, frozen—1½ cups
- ❏ Broccoli, chopped—13 cups
- ❏ Cabbage, red—1 medium head
- ❏ Carrots, baby—4 cups
- ❏ Carrots, chopped—1 cup
- ❏ Carrots, shredded—4 cups

- ❏ Cauliflower—1 medium head
- ❏ Celery—1 bunch
- ❏ Chives—1 bunch
- ❏ Cilantro—1 bunch
- ❏ Cucumber, English—1 small
- ❏ Eggplant—1 large
- ❏ Fennel—1 large bulb
- ❏ Fruit, fresh, chopped—5 cups
- ❏ Garlic—1 head
- ❏ Ginger—1 knot
- ❏ Honeydew melon, chopped—1 cup
- ❏ Kale, chopped—5 cups
- ❏ Lemons—2
- ❏ Limes—2
- ❏ Mango, chopped—1 cup
- ❏ Onions, red—2 small
- ❏ Onions, sweet—1 small, 1 large
- ❏ Onions, yellow—3 medium, 1 large
- ❏ Oranges—4 medium
- ❏ Parsnip—1 medium
- ❏ Parsley—1 bunch
- ❏ Peaches, sliced—1 cup
- ❏ Peppermint—1 bunch
- ❏ Rosemary—1 bunch
- ❏ Salad greens, premixed—6 cups
- ❏ Spinach, baby—2 pounds
- ❏ Sweet potato—1 large
- ❏ Tarragon—1 bunch
- ❏ Tomatoes, cherry—1 cup
- ❏ Tomatoes—2 medium
- ❏ Turnip—1 medium
- ❏ Zucchini—1 small

Poultry, Meat, and Seafood

- ❏ Chicken breast, boneless skinless—12 ounces
- ❏ Chicken breast, grilled—3 ounces
- ❏ Chicken drumsticks and thighs—4 pounds
- ❏ Fish fillet, grilled—3 ounces
- ❏ Tuna, canned in water (low-sodium)—2 (6-ounce) cans
- ❏ Turkey breast, sliced (low-sodium)—3 ounces
- ❏ Turkey, ground, lean—1¼ pounds

Eggs and Dairy Products

- ❑ Cheese, part-skim mozzarella, fresh—1 pound
- ❑ Cheese, part-skim mozzarella, shredded—1½ cups
- ❑ Cheese, reduced-fat blue, crumbled—¼ cup
- ❑ Cheese, reduced-fat cheddar, shredded—½ cup
- ❑ Cheese, reduced-fat cheddar, sliced—4 slices
- ❑ Cheese, reduced-fat Parmesan, shaved—¼ cup
- ❑ Cheese, reduced-fat Parmesan, grated—½ cup
- ❑ Eggs, large—13
- ❑ Egg whites—1 large plus 1 cup
- ❑ Margarine, trans fat–free—3 tablespoons
- ❑ Mayonnaise, reduced-fat—¼ cup
- ❑ Milk, fat-free—1¾ cups
- ❑ Yogurt, fat-free—7½ cups

Grains and Baked Goods

- ❑ Buckwheat, uncooked—¾ cup
- ❑ Buns, whole-wheat, burger—6
- ❑ Bread, whole-wheat—18 slices
- ❑ Breadcrumbs, whole-wheat—2 cups
- ❑ English muffins, whole-wheat—3
- ❑ Flour, whole-wheat, pastry—4 ¾ cups
- ❑ Oats, old-fashioned, uncooked—2 cups
- ❑ Oats, steel-cut, uncooked—1 cup
- ❑ Pasta, whole-wheat, bowtie—12 ounces
- ❑ Quinoa, uncooked—1 cup
- ❑ Rice, uncooked, brown—1 cup
- ❑ Rice cakes, brown—4

Dried, Canned, and Jarred Goods

- ❑ Almonds, sliced—3 tablespoons plus 1 ounce
- ❑ Apple juice, unsweetened—2 cups
- ❑ Applesauce, unsweetened—1 cup
- ❑ Artichoke hearts—1 (14-ounce) can

- ❑ Broth, chicken (low-sodium)—2⅓ cups
- ❑ Broth, vegetable (low-sodium)—8 cups
- ❑ Chocolate chips, reduced-fat—½ cup
- ❑ Seeds, chia—1 tablespoon
- ❑ Seeds, sunflower, toasted—¼ cup
- ❑ Tomato sauce (low-sodium, low-sugar)—1 (24-ounce) jar
- ❑ Walnuts, chopped—2 ounces
- ❑ Yeast, active dry—1 packet

Spices, Sauces, and Pantry Items

- ❑ Baking powder
- ❑ Baking soda
- ❑ Black pepper
- ❑ Dried bay leaf
- ❑ Dried Italian seasoning
- ❑ Dried oregano
- ❑ Dried thyme
- ❑ Ground cinnamon
- ❑ Ground cumin
- ❑ Ground ginger
- ❑ Ground saffron
- ❑ Ground turmeric
- ❑ Honey
- ❑ Mustard, Dijon
- ❑ Mustard, whole-grain
- ❑ Oil, coconut
- ❑ Oil, olive
- ❑ Oil, vegetable
- ❑ Peanut butter
- ❑ Salad dressing, fat-free
- ❑ Salt
- ❑ Sugar, coconut
- ❑ Vanilla extract
- ❑ Vinegar, rice

Week 2 Shopping List (Days 8 to 14)

Fruits and Vegetables

- ❑ Apples—6 medium, 4 large
- ❑ Bananas—1 small, 3 medium
- ❑ Basil—2 cups
- ❑ Bell peppers, green—2 small, 1 medium
- ❑ Bell peppers, red—6 medium
- ❑ Berries, fresh—1 cup
- ❑ Blueberries, fresh—3 cups
- ❑ Broccoli, chopped—1½ cups
- ❑ Carrots, baby—3 cups

- ❏ Cauliflower, chopped—1½ cups
- ❏ Celery—1 bunch
- ❏ Chile, mild green—1 medium
- ❏ Chives—1 bunch
- ❏ Cilantro—2 bunches
- ❏ Corn, frozen—1 cup
- ❏ Cranberries, frozen—12 ounces
- ❏ Cucumbers, English—1 small, 4 medium
- ❏ Fruit, fresh, chopped—5 cups
- ❏ Garlic—1 head
- ❏ Ginger—1 knot
- ❏ Horseradish—1 knot
- ❏ Kale—2 bunches plus 1 cup
- ❏ Lemon—1
- ❏ Limes—5
- ❏ Mangos—2 medium plus 1 cup
- ❏ Mushrooms, sliced—1½ cups
- ❏ Onions, green—7 large
- ❏ Onions, red—3 medium
- ❏ Onions, yellow—3 small, 1 medium, 3 large
- ❏ Parsley—1 bunch
- ❏ Pears—3 medium
- ❏ Peas, sugar snap—1 pound
- ❏ Peppermint—1 bunch
- ❏ Rosemary—1 bunch
- ❏ Salad greens, premixed—6 cups
- ❏ Shallots—3 small
- ❏ Spinach, frozen—1 (10-ounce) package
- ❏ Squash, butternut—2 pounds
- ❏ Tomatoes, Roma—2 large
- ❏ Zucchini—1 small

Poultry, Meat, and Seafood

- ❏ Bacon, turkey, uncooked—2 slices
- ❏ Chicken breast, boneless skinless—1
- ❏ Chicken breast, grilled—3 ounces
- ❏ Ham, sliced (low-sodium)—3 ounces
- ❏ Salmon, boneless—1½ pounds
- ❏ Shrimp, large uncooked, peeled and deveined—1½ pounds
- ❏ Tempeh, chopped—1 cup
- ❏ Tuna, canned in water (low-sodium)—3 ounces

Eggs and Dairy Products

- ❑ Cheese, reduced-fat cheddar, shredded—⅓ cup
- ❑ Cheese, reduced-fat feta, crumbled—8 ounces plus ¾ cup
- ❑ Eggs, large—8
- ❑ Margarine, trans fat–free—3 tablespoons
- ❑ Mayonnaise, reduced-fat—1 tablespoon
- ❑ Milk, fat-free—6¾ cups
- ❑ Yogurt, fat-free—4½ cups

Grains and Baked Goods

- ❑ Bread, whole-wheat—18 slices
- ❑ Cereal, cold whole-grain—1 cup
- ❑ Crackers, whole-wheat—24
- ❑ English muffins, whole-wheat—3
- ❑ Flour, whole-wheat, pastry—2 tablespoons
- ❑ Millet, uncooked—¾ cup
- ❑ Oats, old-fashioned, uncooked—½ cup
- ❑ Oats, steel-cut, uncooked—1 cup
- ❑ Pasta, penne, whole-wheat—12 ounces
- ❑ Pita, whole-wheat—1
- ❑ Quinoa, uncooked—1½ cups
- ❑ Rice, brown, uncooked—1 cup
- ❑ Rice cakes, brown—6

Dried, Canned, and Jarred Goods

- ❑ Almonds, slivered—½ cup
- ❑ Beans, black—1 (15-ounce) can
- ❑ Beans, red kidney—1 (15-ounce) can
- ❑ Bell pepper, red, roasted—¼ cup
- ❑ Broth, chicken (low-sodium)—2 cups
- ❑ Cashews, raw—2 cups
- ❑ Cherries, dried, chopped—1½ cups
- ❑ Chickpeas—1 (15-ounce) can
- ❑ Coconut milk, canned light—1 cup
- ❑ Coconut, unsweetened, shredded—1 cup
- ❑ Cranberries, dried, unsweetened—⅓ cup

- ❏ Dates, pitted Medjool—1 cup
- ❏ Juice, orange, fresh—2 ¼ cups
- ❏ Olives, Kalamata, sliced—¼ cup
- ❏ Pine nuts, raw—⅓ cup
- ❏ Salsa, tomato—1 cup
- ❏ Seeds, sesame, toasted—2 tablespoons
- ❏ Tahini—¼ cup
- ❏ Tomatoes, fresh, diced—1 cup
- ❏ Tomatoes, stewed—2 (14.5-ounce) cans

Spices, Sauces, and Pantry Items

- ❏ Arrowroot powder
- ❏ Black pepper
- ❏ Cayenne
- ❏ Chili powder
- ❏ Dried coriander
- ❏ Dried oregano
- ❏ Garam masala
- ❏ Ground cardamom
- ❏ Ground cinnamon
- ❏ Ground cumin
- ❏ Ground fenugreek
- ❏ Ground ginger
- ❏ Ground saffron
- ❏ Ground turmeric
- ❏ Honey
- ❏ Oil, canola
- ❏ Oil, coconut
- ❏ Oil, olive
- ❏ Oil, sesame
- ❏ Paprika
- ❏ Salad dressing, fat-free
- ❏ Salt
- ❏ Soy sauce, low-sodium
- ❏ Sugar, coconut
- ❏ Vanilla extract
- ❏ Vinegar, rice
- ❏ Vinegar, rice wine

Week 3 Shopping List (Days 15 to 21)

Fruits and Vegetables

- ❏ Apples—4 medium
- ❏ Avocados—4 medium
- ❏ Bananas—5 medium, 1 large
- ❏ Bell peppers, green—2 small
- ❏ Bell peppers, red—1 medium
- ❏ Berries, fresh—3 cups

- ❑ Blackberries, frozen—½ cup
- ❑ Blueberries, fresh—1 cup
- ❑ Blueberries, frozen—½ cup
- ❑ Broccoli florets, frozen—2 cups
- ❑ Carrots, baby—3 cups
- ❑ Carrots, chopped—4 large
- ❑ Carrot, grated—1 cup
- ❑ Cauliflower—1 medium head
- ❑ Celery—1 bunch
- ❑ Chives—1 bunch
- ❑ Cilantro—2 bunches
- ❑ Cucumbers, English—1 small, 1 large
- ❑ Fruit, fresh, chopped—6 cups
- ❑ Garlic—1 head
- ❑ Ginger—1 knot
- ❑ Kale—2 bunches plus 2 cups
- ❑ Lemons—4
- ❑ Limes—6
- ❑ Mango—1 large
- ❑ Mushrooms, crimini, diced—2½ cups
- ❑ Onions, red—1 small, 1 medium
- ❑ Onions, yellow—4 small, 2 large
- ❑ Orange—1 medium
- ❑ Parsley—1 bunch
- ❑ Peaches, frozen, sliced—1 cup
- ❑ Pear—1 medium
- ❑ Peas, sugar snap—1 pound
- ❑ Peppermint—1 bunch
- ❑ Pineapple, frozen, chopped—½ cup
- ❑ Rosemary—1 bunch
- ❑ Sage—1 bunch
- ❑ Salad greens, premixed—4 cups
- ❑ Shallots—3 small
- ❑ Spinach, baby—6 cups
- ❑ Squash, acorn—4 pounds
- ❑ Strawberries, frozen—1 cup
- ❑ Tomatoes, cherry—1 cup
- ❑ Tomatoes, grape—2 cups
- ❑ Tomatoes—8 large

Poultry, Meat, and Seafood

- ❑ Anchovies—6 fillets
- ❑ Chicken breast, boneless skinless—1 pound
- ❑ Chicken breast, grilled—6 ounces
- ❑ Fish fillet, grilled—3 ounces

- ❏ Fish, tilapia—4 (6-ounce) fillets
- ❏ Scallops, uncooked—1½ pounds
- ❏ Shrimp, medium uncooked, peeled and deveined—1½ pounds
- ❏ Turkey, sliced, low-sodium—3 ounces

Eggs and Dairy Products

- ❏ Cheese, part-skim mozzarella, fresh—4 ounces
- ❏ Cheese, reduced-fat cheddar, shredded—½ cup
- ❏ Cheese, reduced-fat Parmesan, grated—1 cup
- ❏ Eggs, large—11
- ❏ Egg whites, large—7
- ❏ Margarine, trans fat–free—3 tablespoons
- ❏ Milk, fat-free—5½ cups
- ❏ Yogurt, fat-free—8 cups

Grains and Baked Goods

- ❏ Amaranth, uncooked—½ cup
- ❏ Bread, whole-wheat—18 slices
- ❏ Breadcrumbs, whole-wheat—¾ cup
- ❏ Crackers, whole-wheat—16
- ❏ Couscous, whole-wheat, uncooked—1 cup
- ❏ English muffins, whole-wheat—2
- ❏ Flour, coconut—2 tablespoons
- ❏ Flour, whole-wheat, pastry—2½ cups
- ❏ Millet, uncooked—¾ cup
- ❏ Oats, old-fashioned, uncooked—3 cups
- ❏ Pasta, spaghetti, whole-wheat—10 ounces
- ❏ Pita, whole-wheat—1
- ❏ Quinoa, uncooked—½ cup
- ❏ Rice, brown, uncooked—2 cups
- ❏ Rice, wild, uncooked—1 cup
- ❏ Rice cakes, brown—6

Dried, Canned, and Jarred Goods

- ❏ Almonds, sliced—¼ cup
- ❏ Almonds, toasted—½ cup
- ❏ Applesauce, unsweetened—1¾ cups

- ❏ Broth, chicken (low-sodium)—11 cups
- ❏ Broth, vegetable (low-sodium)—2¼ cups
- ❏ Coconut, unsweetened, shredded—½ cup
- ❏ Flaxseed, ground—¼ cup
- ❏ Jam—1 tablespoon
- ❏ Juice, apple, unsweetened—1 cup
- ❏ Juice, orange, fresh—1 cup
- ❏ Olives, pitted—¾ cup
- ❏ Peanut butter—2 tablespoons
- ❏ Pecans, chopped—½ cup
- ❏ Seeds, sesame, toasted—2 tablespoons
- ❏ Tahini—¼ cup
- ❏ Walnuts, chopped—1 ounce
- ❏ Wine, dry white—2 tablespoons

Spices, Sauces, and Pantry Items

- ❏ Almond extract
- ❏ Baking powder
- ❏ Baking soda
- ❏ Black pepper
- ❏ Cayenne
- ❏ Chili powder
- ❏ Dried oregano
- ❏ Dried thyme
- ❏ Garlic powder
- ❏ Ground cardamom
- ❏ Ground cinnamon
- ❏ Ground cumin
- ❏ Ground ginger
- ❏ Ground nutmeg
- ❏ Honey
- ❏ Oil, canola
- ❏ Oil, coconut
- ❏ Oil, olive
- ❏ Oil, sesame
- ❏ Onion powder
- ❏ Paprika
- ❏ Salad dressing, fat-free
- ❏ Salt
- ❏ Sugar, coconut
- ❏ Vanilla extract

Week 4 Shopping List (Days 22 to 28)

Fresh Fruits and Vegetables

- ❏ Apples—6 medium, 2 large
- ❏ Arugula—2 cups
- ❏ Avocados—2 medium
- ❏ Banana—1 medium
- ❏ Basil—1 bunch

- ❑ Bell pepper, green—1 medium
- ❑ Berries, fresh—3 cups
- ❑ Broccoli, chopped—6 cups
- ❑ Carrot—1 medium
- ❑ Carrots, baby—4 cups
- ❑ Celery—1 bunch
- ❑ Chives—1 bunch
- ❑ Cilantro—1 bunch
- ❑ Cucumbers, English—1 small, 1 large
- ❑ Fruit, fresh, chopped—8 cups
- ❑ Garlic—1 head
- ❑ Ginger—1 knot
- ❑ Horseradish—1 knot
- ❑ Lemons—8
- ❑ Lettuce—1 head
- ❑ Limes—4
- ❑ Mint—1 bunch
- ❑ Mushrooms, portobello—4 large caps
- ❑ Mushrooms, sliced—2 cups
- ❑ Onions, green—4 large
- ❑ Onions, yellow—3 small, 1 large
- ❑ Oranges—2 medium
- ❑ Pomegranate seeds—3 tablespoons
- ❑ Rosemary—1 bunch
- ❑ Salad greens, premixed—4 cups
- ❑ Shallots, sliced—¾ cup
- ❑ Spinach, baby, fresh—2 pounds plus 6 cups
- ❑ Spinach, frozen—1 (10-ounce) package
- ❑ Sweet potatoes—8 medium, 3 large
- ❑ Thyme, fresh—1 bunch
- ❑ Tomatoes, beefsteak—2 large
- ❑ Tomato, Roma—1 medium
- ❑ Zucchini—3 medium
- ❑ Zucchini, grated—2 cups

Poultry, Meat, and Seafood

- ❑ Chicken breast, grilled—3 ounces
- ❑ Chicken, whole roasting—4½ to 5 pounds
- ❑ Fish fillet, grilled—3 ounces
- ❑ Pork chops, bone-in—4 (6-ounce) chops
- ❑ Tuna, canned in water, low-sodium—3 ounces
- ❑ Turkey, sliced, low-sodium—3 ounces

Eggs and Dairy Products

- ❏ Cheese, part-skim mozzarella, fresh—1 pound
- ❏ Cheese, reduced-fat blue, crumbled—⅔ cup
- ❏ Cheese, reduced-fat Parmesan, shaved—¼ cup
- ❏ Eggs, large—14
- ❏ Egg whites, large—3
- ❏ Margarine, trans fat-free—1 tablespoon
- ❏ Mayonnaise, fat-free—¼ cup
- ❏ Milk, evaporated, fat-free—3½ cups
- ❏ Milk, fat-free—8 cups
- ❏ Milk, sweetened condensed, low-fat—3 tablespoons
- ❏ Sour cream, fat-free—½ cup
- ❏ Yogurt, fat-free—4⅓ cups

Grains and Baked Goods

- ❏ Bread, whole-wheat—2 loaves
- ❏ Breadcrumbs, whole-wheat—1½ cups
- ❏ Buns, whole-wheat, burger—18
- ❏ Cereal, cold whole-grain—1 cup
- ❏ Crackers, whole-wheat—8
- ❏ English muffin, whole-wheat—1
- ❏ Flour, whole-wheat, pastry—2 cups
- ❏ Oats, old-fashioned, uncooked—3 cups
- ❏ Oats, steel-cut, uncooked—1 cup
- ❏ Quinoa, uncooked—½ cup
- ❏ Rice, brown, uncooked—2¾ cups
- ❏ Rice cakes, brown—10

Dried, Canned, and Jarred Goods

- ❏ Applesauce, unsweetened—1¼ cups
- ❏ Basil pesto, fresh—1½ cups
- ❏ Beans, black—1 (15-ounce) can
- ❏ Broth, chicken (low-sodium)—6½ cups
- ❏ Chickpeas—1 (15-ounce) can
- ❏ Cocoa powder, unsweetened—½ cup
- ❏ Coconut milk, light—¼ cup

- ❏ Coconut, shredded unsweetened—½ cup
- ❏ Coconut water—½ cup
- ❏ Juice, apple, unsweetened—1 cup
- ❏ Juice, orange, fresh—½ cup
- ❏ Peanut butter—2 tablespoons
- ❏ Peanuts, chopped—⅓ cup
- ❏ Pumpkin puree—½ cup
- ❏ Raisins, seedless—1⅔ cups
- ❏ Walnuts, chopped—⅓ cup
- ❏ Wine, dry white—1¼ cups

Spices, Sauces, and Pantry Items

- ❏ Baking powder
- ❏ Baking soda
- ❏ Black pepper
- ❏ Cayenne
- ❏ Chili powder
- ❏ Coconut extract
- ❏ Curry powder
- ❏ Ground cardamom
- ❏ Ground cinnamon
- ❏ Ground cumin
- ❏ Ground ginger
- ❏ Ground nutmeg
- ❏ Ground turmeric
- ❏ Honey
- ❏ Maple syrup
- ❏ Mustard, Dijon
- ❏ Oil, canola
- ❏ Oil, olive
- ❏ Salad dressing, fat-free
- ❏ Salt
- ❏ Soy sauce, low-sodium
- ❏ Sugar, coconut
- ❏ Tahini
- ❏ Vanilla extract
- ❏ Vinegar, balsamic

PART II

DASH DIET DETOX RECIPES

CHAPTER 6

BREAKFAST RECIPES

————— • • • • —————

EGGS BAKED IN AVOCADO

Makes 6 servings

3 medium, ripe avocados

6 large eggs

salt and pepper

½ cup reduced-fat shredded cheddar cheese

chopped chives, to serve

1. Preheat the oven to 425°F.

2. Carefully cut the avocados in half, removing the pits but leaving the skin on.

3. Use a small spoon to remove about 2 tablespoons of flesh from the middle of each avocado half, and reserve it for another use.

4. Place the avocado halves cut side up in a glass baking dish.

5. Crack an egg into each avocado half and season lightly with salt and pepper.

6. Bake for 15 to 18 minutes, until the egg is almost set.

7. Sprinkle the eggs with the shredded cheese and bake for another 2 to 3 minutes, until melted.

8. Garnish with chopped chives to serve.

CINNAMON APPLESAUCE BAKED OATMEAL

Makes 9 (1 square) servings

1½ cups fat-free or low-fat milk

½ cup unsweetened applesauce

1 large egg, beaten

2 tablespoons vegetable oil

1 to 2 tablespoons honey

1 teaspoon vanilla extract

2 cups old-fashioned oats, uncooked

1¼ teaspoon ground cinnamon

¼ teaspoon ground ginger

1 teaspoon baking powder

pinch salt

1. Preheat the oven to 375°F. Lightly grease an 8 x 8-inch glass baking dish.

2. Whisk together the milk, applesauce, egg, oil, honey, and vanilla extract in a medium bowl.

3. In a separate medium bowl, stir together the oats, cinnamon, ginger, baking powder, and salt.

4. Stir the dry ingredients into the wet mixture until smooth and well combined.

5. Spread the mixture evenly in the prepared baking dish.

6. Bake for 20 to 25 minutes, until a knife inserted in the center comes out clean.

7. Let cool for 5 minutes, then cut into squares to serve.

VANILLA ALMOND FRENCH TOAST

Makes 8 servings

¾ cup fat-free or low-fat milk

3 large eggs, beaten well

⅓ cup unsweetened applesauce

2 teaspoons vanilla extract

3 tablespoons coconut sugar

1½ teaspoons ground cinnamon

8 slices whole-wheat bread

up to 1 tablespoon maple syrup per slice, to serve

slivered almonds, to serve

1. Preheat a nonstick electric griddle to medium heat.

2. Whisk together the milk, eggs, applesauce, and vanilla extract in a medium bowl.

3. Add the coconut sugar and cinnamon, then whisk until smooth.

4. Soak the slices of bread in the milk mixture, one at a time, until saturated.

5. Place the slices of bread on the griddle in a single layer.

6. Cook the French toast for 2 to 3 minutes on each side, until golden brown.

7. Carefully flip the slices with a plastic spatula and cook for 1 to 2 minutes more, until the underside is browned.

8. Serve hot, drizzled with maple syrup and sprinkled with slivered almonds.

Tips for freezing: *This recipe is great for the whole family, but if you plan to eat one only portion at a time, you can prepare the dish and then freeze the leftovers in individual portions to enjoy throughout the week. Freeze the extra slices in zip-top sandwich bags. To reheat, melt a little margarine in a skillet over medium heat, then add a frozen slice and heat until thawed and warm.*

BROCCOLI CHEESE EGG MUFFINS

Makes 12 servings

canola oil cooking spray

5 cups chopped broccoli florets

6 eggs, beaten well

1 cup liquid egg whites

⅓ cup grated reduced-fat Parmesan cheese

2 tablespoons chopped fresh chives

1 tablespoon minced garlic

½ teaspoon freshly ground pepper

½ cup shredded reduced-fat cheddar cheese

1. Preheat the oven to 350°F. Lightly grease a regular 12-cup muffin pan with cooking spray.

2. Fill a medium saucepan with 1 inch of water, and place a metal steamer insert in the pan.

3. Add the broccoli, then cover and bring to a boil.

4. Steam the broccoli for 4 to 5 minutes, until just tender.

5. In a medium bowl, beat together the eggs, egg whites, Parmesan cheese, chives, garlic, and pepper.

6. Divide the broccoli among the cups of the muffin pan, then fill the cups about three fourths full with the egg mixture.

7. Sprinkle the cheddar cheese over the top.

8. Bake for 18 to 22 minutes, until the egg mixture is just set. Let cool for 5 minutes before serving.

Tips for freezing: *This recipe freezes very well. Simply prepare the egg muffins according to the instructions, then allow the extra muffins to cool to room temperature. Store them all in a zip-top freezer bag and freeze. Reheat in the microwave.*

WHOLE-WHEAT BLUEBERRY PANCAKES

Makes 4 (3-small-pancake) servings

2 cups whole-wheat pastry flour

2¼ teaspoons baking powder

¼ teaspoon ground cinnamon

pinch salt

1¼ cups fat-free or low-fat milk

1 to 2 tablespoons pure maple syrup

1 teaspoon vanilla extract

1 to 1½ cups fresh blueberries

1 tablespoon maple syrup or honey per serving, to serve

1. Preheat a nonstick electric griddle to medium heat.

2. Combine the whole-wheat pastry flour, baking powder, cinnamon, and salt in a medium bowl.

3. In a separate small bowl, whisk together the milk, maple syrup, and vanilla extract until smooth.

4. Whisk the wet ingredients into the dry mixture until smooth and lump-free.

5. Let the batter rest for about 10 minutes at room temperature to thicken.

6. Spoon the batter onto the hot griddle, using about ¼ cup per pancake. Sprinkle a small handful of fresh blueberries into the wet batter of each pancake.

7. Cook for 2 to 3 minutes, until bubbles form in the surface of the pancakes.

8. Carefully flip the pancakes with a plastic spatula and cook for another 1 to 2 minutes, until the underside is lightly browned.

9. Transfer the pancakes to a plate and keep warm. Repeat with the remaining batter.

10. Serve hot, drizzled with maple syrup or honey.

SPINACH AND RED PEPPER FRITTATA

Makes 4 servings

1 tablespoon coconut oil

1 small yellow onion, diced

2 cups chopped baby spinach

1 medium red bell pepper, cored and diced

1 clove garlic, minced

pinch each salt and pepper

3 large eggs plus 5 egg whites, beaten

2 tablespoons fat-free or low-fat milk

¼ cup grated reduced-fat Parmesan cheese

¼ cup chopped cilantro, to serve

1. Preheat the oven to 350°F. Melt the coconut oil in a large, oven-safe skillet over medium heat.

2. Add the onions and spinach and cook for 4 to 6 minutes, until the onion is translucent.

3. Stir in the red pepper, garlic, salt, and pepper; cook for 2 minutes more.

4. Whisk together the eggs, egg whites, milk, and Parmesan cheese in a medium bowl.

5. Pour the mixture into the skillet, stirring until evenly spread.

6. Cook for 2 minutes, until the edges begin to set.

7. Transfer the skillet to the oven and bake for 12 to 15 minutes, until the center is set.

8. Let the frittata cool for about 5 minutes before cutting into wedges.

9. Garnish with chopped cilantro and serve warm.

WHOLE-GRAIN BELGIAN WAFFLES

Makes 8 servings

1 cup whole-wheat pastry flour

2 tablespoons coconut sugar

1½ tablespoons baking powder

½ teaspoon ground cinnamon

pinch salt

1 cup fat-free or low-fat milk

3 tablespoons canola oil

1 egg plus 2 egg whites, beaten well

1 tablespoon maple syrup or honey per waffle, to serve

1. Whisk together the whole-wheat flour, coconut sugar, baking powder, cinnamon, and salt in a medium bowl.

2. Make a well in the dry ingredients, and pour in the milk and oil.

3. Add the egg and egg whites, and stir until just combined.

4. Preheat a Belgian waffle maker according to the instructions, and add about ⅓ cup of batter.

5. Close the waffle iron and cook according to the instructions, until the waffle is crisp and browned.

6. Transfer the waffle to a plate and keep warm; repeat with the remaining batter.

7. Serve the waffles hot, drizzled with maple syrup or honey.

BANANA FLAXSEED MUFFINS

Makes 12 servings

1 cup whole-wheat pastry flour

1 cup old-fashioned oats, uncooked

¼ cup ground flaxseed

1 teaspoon baking soda

1 teaspoon ground cinnamon

pinch ground cardamom

1½ cups mashed banana

½ cup plain fat-free yogurt

¼ cup unsweetened applesauce

2 to 3 tablespoons honey

1½ teaspoons vanilla extract

1. Preheat the oven to 350°F. Line 12 cups of a regular muffin pan with paper liners.

2. Combine the whole-wheat flour, oats, flaxseed, baking soda, cinnamon, and cardamom in a medium bowl.

3. In a separate medium bowl, beat together the banana, yogurt, applesauce, honey, and vanilla extract.

4. Whisk the dry ingredients into the wet mixture in small batches until just combined—the batter will be a little lumpy.

5. Spoon the batter into the muffin cups, filling them about three fourths full.

6. Bake for 22 to 26 minutes, until a knife inserted in the center comes out clean.

7. Let the muffins cool for 5 minutes in the pan, then turn them out onto a wire rack to cool completely.

8. Store extra muffins in an airtight container for up to 2 days.

SAUTÉED SWEET POTATO MUSHROOM HASH

Makes 4 servings

1 tablespoon olive oil

1 large yellow onion, diced

1 teaspoon minced garlic

2 medium sweet potatoes, peeled and diced

2 cups sliced mushrooms

2 tablespoons water

½ teaspoon chili powder

pinch cayenne pepper

pinch each salt and pepper

1 (10-ounce) package frozen spinach, thawed and squeezed to remove moisture

4 large eggs

1. Heat the oil in a large, heavy skillet over medium-high heat.

2. Add the onion and cook for 4 to 5 minutes, until translucent. Stir in the garlic.

3. Cook for 1 minute, until fragrant, then stir in the sweet potatoes and mushrooms.

4. Add the water to the skillet, then cover with the lid and cook for 3 to 4 minutes, until the liquid has cooked off.

5. Remove the lid and spread the mixture evenly on the bottom of the skillet.

6. Sprinkle with chili powder, cayenne, salt, and pepper, then cook for 3 minutes without stirring, until the bottom is browned.

7. Flip the hash using a spatula, then cook for another 2 to 3 minutes, until the sweet potatoes are tender.

8. Stir in the spinach and cook for another 2 minutes, until heated through.

9. Make 4 depressions in the sweet potato hash and crack an egg into each one.

10. Cook for 2 to 3 minutes, until the eggs reach the desired level of doneness. Adjust the seasoning to taste, and serve hot.

———•••••———

CRANBERRY ALMOND BREAKFAST QUINOA

Makes 6 (1-cup) servings

1½ cups quinoa, uncooked

3 cups fat-free or low-fat milk, plus more to serve

3 to 4 tablespoons light brown sugar, packed

⅓ cup unsweetened dried cranberries

⅓ cup slivered almonds

½ teaspoon ground cinnamon

pinch ground ginger

1. Place the quinoa in a bowl and cover with water. Stir by hand, then rinse the quinoa until the water runs clear.

2. Drain the quinoa and set it aside.

3. Pour the milk into a medium saucepan and bring to a boil over medium-high heat.

4. Whisk in the quinoa and return the mixture to a boil.

5. Reduce the heat to medium-low and simmer, covered, for 12 to 15 minutes, until the quinoa has absorbed most of the liquid.

6. Remove the saucepan from the heat, and fluff the quinoa with a fork.

7. Stir in the brown sugar, cranberries, almonds, cinnamon, and ginger, then cover and let rest for 15 minutes.

8. Spoon the quinoa into bowls and serve warm, drizzled with fat-free milk, if desired.

SAUSAGE, SPINACH, AND MUSHROOM OMELET

Makes 1 serving

¼ cup frozen spinach

2 teaspoons olive oil, divided

1 low-sodium turkey breakfast sausage link, sliced thin

¼ cup diced mushrooms

2 large eggs, beaten

1 green onion, sliced thin

1 clove garlic, minced

pinch each salt and pepper

1 to 2 tablespoons chopped parsley

1. Thaw the frozen spinach at room temperature and squeeze as much moisture out of it as you can.

2. Heat 1 teaspoon of the oil in a small skillet over medium heat.

3. Add the sausage, mushrooms, and spinach and cook for 2 to 3 minutes, stirring occasionally, until the sausage is heated through.

4. Spoon the mixture off into a small bowl and reheat the skillet with the remaining 1 teaspoon oil.

5. Whisk together the eggs, green onion, garlic, salt, and pepper in a small bowl.

6. Pour the egg mixture into the skillet, tilting the pan to spread the mixture.

7. Cook for 2 minutes, until the edges of the egg mixture begin to set, then tilt the pan again, spreading the uncooked egg.

8. Cook for another 30 to 60 seconds, until the egg mixture is almost set.

9. Spoon the sausage, spinach, and mushroom mixture over half the omelet. Sprinkle with the parsley.

10. Fold the empty half of the omelet over the filling.

11. Cook for 30 to 60 seconds more, until the egg mixture is set, then slide onto a plate to serve.

BUTTERMILK WAFFLES WITH HONEY

Makes 8 servings

1 cup whole-wheat pastry flour

1½ tablespoons baking powder

pinch salt

1 cup low-fat buttermilk

2 tablespoons canola oil

2 tablespoons honey

½ teaspoon vanilla extract

1 egg plus 2 egg whites, beaten well

1 tablespoons honey or maple syrup per waffle, to serve

1. Whisk together the whole-wheat flour, baking powder, and salt in a medium bowl.

2. Make a well in the dry ingredients and pour in the buttermilk, oil, honey, and vanilla extract.

3. Add the egg and egg whites, and stir until just combined.

4. Preheat a Belgian waffle maker according to the instructions and add about ⅓ cup of batter.

5. Close the waffle iron and cook according to the instructions until the waffle is crisp and browned.

6. Transfer the waffle to a plate and keep warm. Repeat with the remaining batter.

7. Serve the waffles hot, drizzled with honey or maple syrup.

MINI MUSHROOM AND ONION QUICHES

Makes 12 servings

canola oil cooking spray

1½ cups diced mushrooms

1 small Vidalia onion, diced

6 eggs, beaten well

1 cup liquid egg whites

1 green onion, sliced thin

1 teaspoon minced garlic

½ teaspoon freshly ground pepper

½ cup grated reduced-fat Parmesan cheese

1. Preheat the oven to 350°F. Lightly grease a regular 12-cup muffin pan with cooking spray.

2. Combine the mushrooms and onion in a medium bowl, stirring well.

3. In a separate medium bowl, beat together the eggs, egg whites, green onion, garlic, and pepper.

4. Divide the mushroom and onion mixture among the cups of the muffin pan, then fill the cups about three fourths full with the egg mixture.

5. Sprinkle the Parmesan cheese over the top.

6. Bake for 18 to 22 minutes, until the egg mixture is just set. Let cool for 5 minutes before serving.

Tips for freezing: *This recipe freezes very well. Simply prepare the quiches according to the instructions, then allow the extra ones to cool to room temperature. Store them all in a zip-top freezer bag and freeze. Reheat in the microwave.*

CHOCO-COCONUT FRENCH TOAST

Makes 8 servings

¾ cup fat-free or low-fat milk

3 large eggs, beaten well

¼ cup canned light coconut milk

1 teaspoon coconut extract

3 tablespoons coconut sugar

2 tablespoons unsweetened cocoa powder

8 slices whole-wheat bread

up to 1 tablespoon honey per slice, to serve

shredded unsweetened coconut, to serve

1. Preheat a nonstick electric griddle to medium heat.

2. Whisk together the milk, eggs, coconut milk, and coconut extract in a medium bowl.

3. Add the coconut sugar and cocoa powder, then whisk until smooth.

4. Soak the slices of bread in the milk mixture, one at a time, until saturated.

5. Place the slices of bread on the griddle in a single layer.

6. Cook the French toast for 2 to 3 minutes on each side, until golden brown.

7. Carefully flip the slices with a plastic spatula and cook for 1 to 2 minutes more, until the underside is browned.

8. Serve the French toast hot, drizzled with honey and sprinkled with shredded coconut.

Tips for freezing: *If you plan to eat only one portion at a time, you can prepare the dish and then freeze the leftovers in individual portions to enjoy throughout the week. Freeze the extra slices in zip-top sandwich bags. To reheat, melt a little margarine in a skillet over medium heat, then add a frozen slice and heat until thawed and warm.*

CINNAMON BANANA PANCAKES

Makes 4 (3-small-pancake) servings

2 cups whole-wheat pastry flour

1¾ teaspoons baking powder

1¾ teaspoons baking soda

1 teaspoon ground cinnamon

¼ teaspoon ground ginger

pinch salt

1¾ cups fat-free or low-fat milk

2 tablespoons canola oil

1 to 2 tablespoons honey

2 large eggs, beaten well

2 medium, ripe bananas, peeled and mashed

1 tablespoon maple syrup or honey per serving, to serve

1. Preheat a nonstick electric griddle to medium heat.

2. Combine the whole-wheat pastry flour, baking powder, baking soda, cinnamon, ginger, and salt in a medium bowl.

3. In a separate medium bowl, whisk together the milk, canola oil, honey, and eggs until smooth.

4. Fold in the mashed banana, then whisk the wet ingredients into the dry mixture until smooth and lump-free.

5. Spoon the batter onto the hot griddle, using about ¼ cup per pancake.

6. Cook for 2 to 3 minutes, until bubbles form on the surface of the pancakes.

7. Carefully flip the pancakes with a plastic spatula and cook for another 1 to 2 minutes, until the underside is lightly browned.

8. Transfer the pancakes to a plate and keep warm. Repeat with the remaining batter.

9. Serve hot, drizzled with maple syrup or honey.

ROASTED RED PEPPER AND FETA OMELET

Makes 1 serving

1 teaspoon olive oil

2 large eggs, beaten

1 green onion, sliced thin

pinch each salt and pepper

¼ cup chopped roasted red bell pepper

2 to 3 tablespoons reduced-fat feta cheese crumbles

1 teaspoon grated fresh horseradish

pinch dried oregano

1. Heat the oil in a small skillet over medium heat.

2. Whisk together the eggs, green onion, salt, and pepper in a small bowl.

3. Pour the egg mixture into the skillet, tilting the pan to spread the egg.

4. Cook for 2 minutes, until the edges of the egg mixture begin to set, then tilt the pan again, spreading the uncooked egg.

5. Cook for another 30 to 60 seconds, until the egg mixture is almost set.

6. Spread the roasted red pepper and feta cheese over half the omelet. Sprinkle with the horseradish and oregano.

7. Fold the empty half of the omelet over the filling.

8. Cook for 30 to 60 seconds more, until the egg mixture is set, then slide onto a plate to serve.

BAKED EGGS IN A BASKET

Makes 4 servings

2 slices low-sodium turkey bacon

1 tablespoon trans fat–free margarine

4 slices whole-wheat bread

4 large eggs

⅓ cup reduced-fat shredded cheddar cheese

salt and pepper

1. Preheat the oven to 400°F.

2. Cook the bacon in a large, oven-safe skillet over medium-high heat until crisp.

3. Remove the bacon to paper towels to drain, and then crumble and set aside.

4. Spread some of the margarine over one side of each slice of bread.

5. Use a 3-inch round cookie cutter to cut out the middle of each slice of bread.

6. Place the slices of bread in the hot skillet, margarine side down, and crack an egg into the hole in each slice.

7. If there is room in the skillet, add the cut-outs from the bread slices.

8. Sprinkle the cheese and crumbled bacon over the egg, and season with lightly with salt and pepper.

9. Transfer the skillet to the oven and bake for 5 minutes, or until the egg whites are set.

10. Serve hot, with the cut-outs to dip in the egg yolk.

BAKED CRANBERRY PECAN OATMEAL

Makes 9 (1 square) servings

1½ cups fat-free or low-fat milk

½ cup unsweetened applesauce

1 large egg, beaten

2 tablespoons olive oil

1 teaspoon almond extract

2 cups old-fashioned oats, uncooked

½ cup unsweetened dried cranberries

¼ cup finely chopped pecans

1 teaspoon baking powder

pinch ground ginger

pinch salt

2 tablespoons light brown sugar

1. Preheat the oven to 375°F. Lightly grease an 8 x 8-inch glass baking dish.

2. Whisk together the milk, applesauce, egg, oil, and almond extract in a medium bowl.

3. In a separate medium bowl, stir together the oats, cranberries, pecans, baking powder, ginger, and salt.

4. Stir the dry ingredients into the wet mixture until smooth and well combined.

5. Spread the mixture evenly in the prepared baking dish.

6. Bake for 20 to 25 minutes, until a knife inserted in the center comes out clean.

7. Turn on the broiler. Sprinkle the brown sugar over the oatmeal and place under the broiler for 2 to 3 minutes, until the sugar is bubbling.

8. Let cool for 5 minutes, then cut into 9 squares to serve.

GREEK-STYLE CRUSTLESS QUICHE

Makes 4 servings

1 tablespoon coconut oil

1 small red onion, diced

2 cups chopped baby spinach

½ cup diced tomatoes

¼ cup chopped roasted red bell pepper

¼ cup chopped black olives

2 teaspoons minced garlic

pinch each salt and pepper

3 large eggs plus 5 egg whites, beaten

2 tablespoons fat-free or low-fat milk

½ cup feta cheese crumbles

2 tablespoons chopped fresh mint, to serve

1. Preheat the oven to 350°F. Melt the coconut oil in a large, oven-safe skillet over medium heat.

2. Add the onions and spinach, then cook for 4 to 6 minutes, until the onion is translucent and the spinach is wilted.

3. Stir in the tomatoes, roasted red pepper, olives, and garlic.

4. Season with a pinch each of salt and pepper, then cook for 2 minutes more.

5. Whisk together the eggs, egg whites, and milk in a medium bowl.

6. Pour the egg mixture into the skillet, stirring until evenly spread.

7. Cook for 2 minutes, until the edges begin to set, then sprinkle with feta cheese.

8. Transfer the skillet to the oven and bake for 12 to 15 minutes, until the center is set.

9. Let the quiche cool for about 5 minutes before cutting into wedges to serve. Garnish with the mint.

HONEY RAISIN FRENCH TOAST

Makes 8 servings

¾ cup fat-free or low-fat milk

3 large eggs, beaten well

¼ cup unsweetened applesauce

2 tablespoons honey

1 teaspoon vanilla extract

1½ teaspoons ground cinnamon

½ teaspoon ground nutmeg

pinch ground ginger

8 slices whole-wheat bread

1 tablespoons honey or maple syrup per slice, to serve

2 tablespoons seedless raisins, to serve

1. Preheat a nonstick electric griddle to medium heat.

2. Whisk together the milk, eggs, applesauce, honey, and vanilla extract in a medium bowl.

3. Add the cinnamon, nutmeg, and ginger, then whisk until smooth.

4. Soak the slices of bread in the milk mixture, one at a time, until saturated.

5. Place the slices of bread on the griddle in a single layer.

6. Cook the French toast for 2 to 3 minutes on each side, until golden brown.

7. Carefully flip the slices with a plastic spatula and cook for 1 to 2 minutes more, until the underside is browned.

8. Serve hot, drizzled with honey or maple syrup and sprinkled with raisins.

Tips for freezing: *To enjoy one portion at a time, you can prepare the French toast and then freeze the leftovers in individual portions to have throughout the week. To reheat, melt a little margarine in a skillet over medium heat, then add a frozen slice and heat until thawed and warm.*

SIMPLE BUTTERMILK PANCAKES

Makes 6 (2-small-pancake) servings

1½ cups whole-wheat pastry flour

1¾ teaspoons baking powder

½ teaspoon baking soda

½ teaspoon ground cinnamon

pinch of salt

1½ cups low-fat buttermilk

2 tablespoons canola oil

1 to 2 tablespoons granulated sugar

1 large egg, beaten

1 teaspoon vanilla extract

1 tablespoons maple syrup or honey per serving, to serve

1. Combine the whole-wheat pastry flour, baking powder, baking soda, and cinnamon in a medium bowl.

2. In a separate medium bowl, whisk together the buttermilk, canola oil, sugar, egg, and vanilla extract until smooth.

3. Whisk the wet ingredients into the dry mixture until smooth and lump-free.

4. Preheat a nonstick electric griddle to medium heat.

5. Let the batter rest for 10 to 15 minutes at room temperature to thicken.

6. Spoon the batter onto the hot griddle, using about ¼ cup per pancake. Cook for 2 to 3 minutes, until bubbles form on the surface of the pancakes.

7. Carefully flip the pancakes with a plastic spatula and cook for another 1 to 2 minutes, until the underside is lightly browned.

8. Transfer the pancakes to a plate and keep warm. Repeat with the remaining batter.

9. Serve the pancakes hot, drizzled with maple syrup or honey.

WHOLE-WHEAT PUMPKIN PANCAKES

Makes 8 (2-pancake) servings

3 cups whole-wheat pastry flour

2½ tablespoons baking powder

2 teaspoons ground cinnamon

½ teaspoon ground nutmeg

pinch salt

2½ cups low-fat buttermilk

1¼ cups pumpkin puree

¼ cup canola oil

2 large eggs plus 1 egg white

1 tablespoon maple syrup or honey per serving, to serve

1. Preheat an electric griddle to medium heat.

2. Whisk together the whole-wheat pastry flour, baking powder, cinnamon, nutmeg, and salt in a large bowl.

3. In a separate medium bowl, beat together the buttermilk, pumpkin puree, oil, eggs, and egg white until smooth.

4. Beat the wet ingredients into the dry mixture until just incorporated.

5. Spoon the batter onto the preheated griddle, using about ¼ cup of batter per pancake.

6. Cook for 2 to 3 minutes, until bubbles appear in the surface of the batter.

7. Carefully flip the pancakes, using a plastic spatula, and cook for another 1 to 2 minutes, until the underside is lightly browned.

8. Transfer the pancakes to a plate and keep warm, then repeat with the remaining batter.

9. Serve the pancakes hot, drizzled with maple syrup or honey.

WHOLE-GRAIN WALNUT PECAN MUESLI

Makes 8 (½-cup) servings

1½ cups old-fashioned oats, uncooked

1½ cups plain fat-free yogurt

¾ cup fat-free or low-fat milk

pinch salt

1 cup seedless raisins

½ cup toasted walnuts, chopped

½ cup toasted pecans, chopped

½ teaspoon ground cinnamon

honey, to serve

1. Combine the oats, yogurt, milk, and salt in a medium bowl.

2. Cover the bowl with plastic and chill in the refrigerator for 8 to 12 hours or overnight.

3. Stir in the raisins, walnuts, pecans, and cinnamon.

4. Spoon the muesli into bowls and drizzle with honey to serve.

CHERRY CINNAMON OVERNIGHT OATS

Makes 4 servings

2 cups fat-free or low-fat milk, plus more to serve

2 cups water

1 cup steel-cut oats, uncooked

½ cup dried cherries, chopped

1 tablespoon honey

½ to 1 teaspoon ground cinnamon

pinch ground ginger

pinch salt

1. Whisk together the milk, water, and steel-cut oats in a slow cooker.

2. Stir in the cherries, honey, cinnamon, ginger, and salt until well combined.

3. Cover the slow cooker and cook on low heat for 8 to 9 hours, or overnight.

4. Spoon the oatmeal into bowls and drizzle with fat-free milk to serve.

HOMEMADE TURKEY SAUSAGE PATTIES

Makes 6 (2-patty) servings

1 pound lean ground turkey

1 small yellow onion, diced fine

2 teaspoons dried sage

1½ teaspoons fennel seed

1 teaspoon garlic powder

¼ teaspoon ground cumin

pinch each salt and pepper

1 tablespoon olive oil

1. Combine the turkey, onion, sage, fennel seed, garlic powder, and cumin in a large bowl, and season with a pinch each of salt and pepper.

2. Mix the ingredients well, then shape by hand into 3-inch patties.

3. Heat the oil in a large, heavy skillet over medium-high heat.

4. Add the patties and cook for 2 to 3 minutes on each side, until browned and no longer pink in the middle, and serve hot.

LEMON POPPY SEED MUFFINS

Makes 12 servings

1½ cups whole-wheat pastry flour

¼ cup poppy seeds

1¼ teaspoons baking powder

½ teaspoon baking soda

pinch salt

grated zest and juice of 2 lemons

½ cup coconut sugar

⅓ cup unsweetened applesauce

¾ cup plain fat-free yogurt

2 large eggs, beaten

1 teaspoon vanilla extract

1. Preheat the oven to 375°F. Line 12 cups of a regular muffin pan with paper liners.

2. Combine the whole-wheat flour, poppy seeds, baking powder, baking soda, and salt in a medium bowl.

3. In a small bowl, stir together the lemon zest and coconut sugar, then whisk into the dry ingredients.

4. In a separate medium bowl, beat together the applesauce, yogurt, eggs, lemon juice, and vanilla extract.

5. Whisk the wet ingredients into the dry mixture in small batches until just combined.

6. Spoon the batter into the prepared muffin cups, filling them about three fourths full.

7. Bake for 15 to 18 minutes, until a knife inserted in the center comes out clean.

8. Let the muffins cool in the pan for 5 minutes, then turn out onto a wire rack to cool completely.

9. Store extra muffins in an airtight container for up to 2 days.

SPINACH AND EGG STUFFED PEPPERS

Makes 6 (½-pepper) servings

3 large bell peppers, assorted colors

1 teaspoon olive oil

1 small yellow onion, diced

1 clove garlic, minced

4 cups chopped baby spinach

pinch each salt and pepper

6 large eggs

½ cup reduced-fat shredded cheddar cheese

chopped chives, to serve

1. Preheat the oven to 400°F.

2. Bring a large pot of water to a boil and add the peppers.

3. Blanch the peppers for about 60 seconds, then plunge them into an ice bath to stop the cooking.

4. Let the peppers cool slightly, then slice them in half lengthwise and remove the seeds and ribs.

5. Arrange the peppers cut side up in an 8 x 8-inch square glass baking dish.

6. Heat the oil in a large skillet over medium heat.

7. Add the onion and garlic and cook for 5 to 6 minutes, until the onion is translucent.

8. Stir in the spinach and season with salt and pepper.

9. Cook for 2 to 3 minutes, until the spinach is wilted, then divide the mixture among the peppers in the baking dish.

10. Crack an egg into each pepper and sprinkle with cheese.

11. Bake the peppers for 10 to 12 minutes, until the eggs are set and the peppers are tender.

12. Serve hot, garnished with chopped chives.

TOMATO BASIL EGG WHITE OMELET

Makes 1 serving

1 teaspoon olive oil, divided

1 medium Roma tomato, cored and diced

2 to 3 tablespoons diced yellow onion

3 large egg whites, beaten

1 tablespoon chopped chives

pinch each salt and pepper

4 to 6 fresh basil leaves, coarsely chopped

1. Heat ½ teaspoon of the oil in a small skillet over medium heat.

2. Add the tomato and onion and cook for 2 to 3 minutes, stirring occasionally, until the onion is translucent.

3. Spoon the mixture into a bowl and reheat the skillet with the remaining ½ teaspoon oil.

4. Whisk together the egg whites, chives, salt, and pepper in a small bowl.

5. Pour the egg mixture into the skillet, tilting the pan to spread the egg.

6. Cook for 2 minutes, until the edges of the egg mixture begin to set, then tilt the pan again, spreading the uncooked egg.

7. Let the egg whites cook for another 30 to 60 seconds, until almost set.

8. Spoon the tomato and onion mixture over half the omelet and sprinkle with the basil.

9. Fold the empty half of the omelet over the filling.

10. Cook for 30 to 60 seconds more, until the egg mixture is set, then slide onto a plate to serve.

HAM AND CHEESE EGG CUPS

Makes 12 (1-egg-cup) servings

canola oil cooking spray

6 eggs, beaten well

1 cup liquid egg whites

⅓ cup shredded part-skim mozzarella cheese

½ teaspoon freshly ground pepper

2 cups diced low-sodium ham

½ cup shredded reduced-fat cheddar cheese

1. Preheat the oven to 350°F. Lightly grease a regular 12-cup muffin pan with cooking spray.

2. In a medium bowl, beat together the eggs, egg whites, mozzarella cheese, and pepper.

3. Divide the diced ham among the cups of the muffin pan, then fill them about three fourths full with the egg mixture.

4. Sprinkle the cheddar cheese over the top of the egg mixture.

5. Bake for 18 to 22 minutes, until the egg is just set. Let cool for 5 minutes before serving.

Tips for freezing: *This recipe freezes very well. Simply prepare the egg cups according to the instructions, then allow the extra cups to cool to room temperature. Store them all in a zip-tip freezer bag and freeze. Reheat in the microwave.*

PEANUT BUTTER BANANA OATMEAL BAKE

Makes 9 (1 square) servings

1½ cups fat-free or low-fat milk

2 small bananas, peeled and mashed

1 large egg, beaten

2 tablespoons olive oil

2 tablespoons low-sodium, smooth peanut butter

1 teaspoon vanilla extract

2 cups old-fashioned oats, uncooked

1 teaspoon baking powder

½ teaspoon ground cinnamon

pinch salt

1. Preheat the oven to 375°F. Lightly grease an 8 x 8-inch square glass baking dish.

2. Whisk together the milk, banana, egg, oil, peanut butter, and vanilla extract in a medium bowl.

3. In a separate medium bowl, stir together the oats, baking powder, cinnamon, and salt.

4. Stir the dry ingredients into the wet mixture until smooth and well combined.

5. Spread the mixture evenly in the prepared baking dish.

6. Bake for 22 to 26 minutes, until a knife inserted in the center comes out clean.

7. Let cool for 5 minutes, then cut into 9 squares to serve.

CHAPTER 7

LUNCH RECIPES

● ● ● ●

CRANBERRY FETA CHICKEN SANDWICHES

Makes 4 servings

1 (12-ounce bag) frozen cranberries

1 cup fresh orange juice

¼ cup honey

1 teaspoon ground cinnamon

8 slices whole-wheat bread, toasted

1 boneless, skinless chicken breast, cooked and sliced thin

8 ounces reduced-fat feta cheese, sliced

1. Combine the cranberries, orange juice, honey, and cinnamon in a medium saucepan.

2. Bring the mixture to a boil, reduce the heat, and simmer for about 10 minutes, until thick.

3. Remove from the heat and let cool to room temperature.

4. Lay half of the slices of toasted bread out flat, and top each one with sliced chicken.

5. Add a slice of feta cheese to each slice and top with a few tablespoons of the cranberry sauce.

6. Top each with a second slice of toasted bread. Cut the sandwiches in half and serve immediately.

ROASTED ROOT VEGETABLE AND CAULIFLOWER SOUP

Makes 6 to 8 (1-cup) servings

1 medium head cauliflower, cut into florets

1 large yellow onion, quartered

1 cup baby carrots

1 medium parsnip, peeled and chopped

1 medium turnip, peeled and chopped

2 to 3 tablespoons olive oil

pinch each salt and pepper

4 cups low-sodium vegetable broth

1 cup water

1 bay leaf

½ teaspoon ground turmeric

pinch ground cumin

1. Preheat the oven to 400°F. Line a rimmed baking sheet with foil.

2. Spread the cauliflower, onion, carrots, parsnips, and turnips on the baking sheet in a single layer.

3. Drizzle with the olive oil and season with a pinch of salt and pepper.

4. Roast the vegetables for 18 to 25 minutes, until fork tender.

5. Remove the vegetables from the oven and let cool slightly before chopping them coarsely.

6. Combine the vegetable broth, water, and roasted vegetables in a large stockpot over high heat.

7. Add the bay leaf, turmeric, and cumin, then bring to a boil.

8. Reduce the heat and simmer, uncovered, for 18 to 20 minutes, until the vegetables are very tender.

9. Remove the bay leaf, then puree the soup using an immersion blender or in batches using a food processor or high-speed blender.

10. Adjust the seasonings to taste. Serve hot.

—— • • • • ——

OPEN-FACED TUNA MELT

Makes 2 servings

2 (6-ounce) cans low-sodium tuna in water, drained

1 small stalk celery, diced

2 tablespoons minced red onion

1 teaspoon chopped parsley

¼ cup fat-free mayonnaise

1 tablespoon Dijon mustard

1 teaspoon lemon juice

pinch each salt and pepper

2 tablespoons trans fat–free margarine

4 slices whole-wheat bread

4 slices reduced-fat cheddar cheese

1. Preheat the broiler in your oven to high heat.

2. Flake the tuna into a medium bowl and stir in the celery, red onion, and parsley.

3. Add the mayonnaise, mustard, and lemon juice, then season with a pinch each of salt and pepper.

4. Spread the margarine on one side of each slice of whole-wheat bread. Place the slices of bread, margarine side up, on a baking sheet.

5. Top the bread with the tuna salad and a slice of cheddar cheese.

6. Slide the tuna melts under the broiler.

7. Broil for 3 to 5 minutes, until the cheese is melted and the bread is toasted, and serve hot.

BAKED ROOT VEGETABLE CAKES

Makes 8 (2-vegetable-cake) servings

2 cups grated peeled russet potatoes

2 cups grated peeled sweet potatoes

3 large parsnips, peeled and grated

2 large carrots, peeled and grated

1 small yellow onion, diced

2 tablespoons fresh chopped parsley

2 large eggs, beaten well

¼ cup whole-wheat pastry flour

¼ teaspoon ground cardamom

pinch each salt and pepper

1. Preheat the oven to 400°F. Line a rimmed baking sheet with parchment.

2. Combine the potatoes, sweet potatoes, parsnips, and carrots in a large bowl.

3. Stir in the onion, parsley, eggs, flour, and cardamom, and season with a pinch each of salt and pepper.

4. Drop spoonfuls of the mixture onto the prepared baking sheet, using about ¼ cup per cake.

5. Flatten the cakes slightly by hand, then bake for 10 minutes.

6. Flip the vegetable cakes and bake for another 10 minutes, until the outside is crisped and brown, and serve hot.

CHICKPEA SUMMER SALAD

Makes 4 to 6 (1-cup) servings

3 (15-ounce) cans chickpeas, rinsed and drained

3 ears corn on the cob, grilled, kernels cut from the cob

3 cups grape tomatoes, quartered

4 to 5 green onions, sliced thin

¼ cup chopped cilantro

2 tablespoons chopped chives

pinch each salt and pepper

¼ cup olive oil

2½ tablespoons red wine vinegar

grated zest and juice of 1 lime

2 tablespoons honey

1 tablespoon minced garlic

1. Combine the chickpeas, corn, tomatoes, and green onions in a large bowl.

2. Add the cilantro and chives and toss to combine, then season with a pinch each of salt and pepper.

3. In a small saucepan, whisk together the oil, vinegar, lime juice, and honey.

4. Stir in the lime zest and garlic, then cook over low heat for 5 minutes, stirring often.

5. Let the dressing cool for 5 minutes then pour the dressing over the salad and toss to coat.

6. Cover the bowl with plastic and chill for 1 hour before serving.

BARLEY SOUP WITH WHITE BEANS AND KALE

Makes 6 to 8 (1-cup) servings

3 cups water or vegetable broth

1 cup hulled barley, uncooked

1 tablespoon olive oil

1 medium yellow onion, chopped

1 tablespoon minced garlic

5 cups chicken broth

2 (15-ounce) cans white cannellini beans, rinsed and drained

1 (14.5-ounce) can diced tomatoes

1 tablespoon chopped fresh rosemary

½ teaspoon chopped fresh thyme

¼ teaspoon chopped fresh tarragon

pinch ground cardamom

2 to 3 cups chopped kale, large stems removed

1 tablespoon lemon juice

pinch each salt and pepper

1. Combine the water and barley in a large saucepan over high heat.

2. Bring the water to a boil, reduce the heat, and simmer for 40 to 45 minutes, until tender.

3. Drain the barley and set it aside.

4. Heat the oil in a stockpot over medium heat.

5. Stir in the onion and garlic and cook for 5 to 6 minutes, until the onion is translucent.

6. Add the chicken broth, white beans, tomatoes, herbs, and cardamom, then bring to a boil.

7. Reduce the heat and simmer the soup for about 30 minutes.

8. Stir in the cooked barley along with the kale and simmer for a few minutes, until the kale is just wilted.

9. Whisk in the lemon juice and season with a pinch each of salt and pepper. Serve hot.

   To cook your own beans: Rinse 8 ounces dried white cannellini beans, and soak in water to cover overnight. Drain the beans well, then transfer them to a large saucepan and cover with 2 inches of cold water. Bring to a boil, reduce the heat, and simmer, covered, for up to 1½ hours, until tender. Use as directed.

TURKEY BLTA SANDWICHES

Makes 4 servings

6 slices low-sodium turkey bacon

8 slices whole-wheat bread, toasted

1 romaine heart, leaves torn to fit bread

1 large beefsteak tomato, sliced

1 ripe avocado, pitted and sliced thin

pinch each salt and pepper (optional)

¼ cup fat-free mayonnaise

1. Cook the turkey bacon in a large skillet over medium heat until crisp.

2. Drain the bacon on paper towels, then break the slices in half.

3. Lay the slices of toasted whole-wheat bread out flat.

4. Top half of the slices with a leaf or two of romaine followed by a slice of tomato.

5. Add 3 half-pieces of bacon on each sandwich, along with a few slices of avocado. Season with a pinch each of salt and pepper, if desired.

6. Spread the mayonnaise over the remaining slices of toasted bread and use them to top off the sandwiches.

7. Cut the sandwiches in half and serve immediately.

ROASTED ACORN SQUASH SOUP
WITH TOASTED PECANS

Makes 6 to 8 (1-cup) servings

3 to 4 pounds acorn squash, peeled, seeded, and chopped

4 large carrots, peeled and chopped

1 large yellow onion, chopped

1 tablespoon minced garlic

olive oil, as needed

2 tablespoons light brown sugar

2 tablespoons trans fat–free margarine

½ cup coarsely chopped pecans

¼ teaspoon ground cinnamon, plus more for the pecans

6 cups low-sodium chicken broth

1 teaspoon chopped fresh sage

salt and pepper

1. Preheat the oven to 375°F. Line a rimmed baking sheet with foil.

2. Spread the squash, carrots, onion, and garlic on the baking sheet in a single layer.

3. Drizzle with olive oil, then season salt and pepper.

4. Toss the vegetables with the brown sugar, then roast for 20 minutes.

5. Turn the vegetables once, and roast for another 20 to 25 minutes, until fork-tender.

6. While the vegetables are roasting, melt the margarine in a large skillet over medium heat.

7. Add the pecans and toss to coat with the margarine, then sprinkle with cinnamon to taste and a pinch each of salt and pepper.

8. Cook the pecans for 2 to 3 minutes, until toasted, stirring often to keep them from burning.

9. Transfer the pecans to paper towels to drain and cool.

10. Bring the chicken broth to a boil in a large stockpot, then remove from the heat.

11. Stir the roasted vegetables into the broth along with the sage and ¼ teaspoon cinnamon.

12. Puree the soup using an immersion blender or in batches using a food processor.

13. Spoon the soup into bowls and garnish with the toasted pecans.

CHILLED AVOCADO SOUP

Makes 6 to 8 (1-cup) servings

4 large, ripe avocados, pitted and chopped

4 cups low-sodium chicken or vegetable broth

2 medium shallots, diced

1 cup fat-free or low-fat milk

1 tablespoon cooking sherry

pinch each salt and pepper

fat-free sour cream, to serve

ground saffron, to serve

1. Combine the avocado, chicken broth, and shallots in a food processor.

2. Process until smooth and well combined, then pulse in the milk and sherry.

3. Season with a pinch each of salt and pepper and blend until smooth.

4. Transfer the mixture to a bowl, cover with plastic, and chill for at least 6 hours, until cold.

5. Spoon the soup into bowls and garnish with a dollop of fat-free sour cream.

6. Sprinkle each bowl with a pinch of ground saffron to serve.

FRIED SUMMER SQUASH FRITTERS

Makes 6 (3-fritter) servings

1½ pounds summer squash, peeled

1 medium yellow onion, diced

1 large egg plus 1 egg white, whisked

1¼ teaspoons garlic powder

pinch cayenne (optional)

olive oil, as needed

salt and pepper

1. Grate or shred the summer squash using the shredding blade attachment of a food processor.

2. Spread the grated squash on a clean towel and sprinkle lightly with salt.

3. Let the squash rest for 15 minutes, then roll up the towel and wring it out, squeezing as much moisture from the squash as possible.

4. Transfer the squash to a medium bowl and stir in the onion, egg and egg white, and garlic powder.

5. Stir the mixture well, seasoning with a pinch each of cayenne, salt, and pepper.

6. Heat enough oil to cover the bottom of a large skillet over medium-high heat.

7. Spoon the squash mixture into the skillet, using about ¼ cup per fritter.

8. Cook for 4 to 5 minutes without moving, until the bottoms are browned.

9. Carefully flip the fritters and cook for 3 to 4 minutes on the other side, until browned.

10. Drain the fritters on paper towels and serve hot.

SOUTHWESTERN THREE-BEAN SALAD

Makes 10 to 12 (1-cup) servings

1 (15-ounce) can black beans, rinsed and drained

1 (15-ounce) can red kidney beans, rinsed and drained

1 (15-ounce) can chickpeas, rinsed and drained

1 medium red onion, diced small

1 cup diced celery

1 cup diced ripe tomatoes

1 cup frozen corn kernels, thawed

1 cup fresh tomato salsa

¼ cup chopped cilantro

¼ cup lime juice

2 tablespoons olive oil

1½ teaspoons chili powder

1 teaspoon ground cumin

pinch cayenne

pinch salt

1. Combine the black beans, kidney beans, and chickpeas in a large bowl.

2. Stir in the onion, celery, tomato, and corn.

3. In a small bowl, whisk together the salsa, cilantro, lime juice, olive oil, chili powder, cumin, cayenne, and salt.

4. Toss the salad with the dressing, then cover and chill for 2 to 4 hours before serving.

To cook your own beans: *Rinse 4 ounces each of dried black beans, red kidney beans, and chickpeas, and soak in water to cover overnight. Drain the beans well, then transfer them to a large saucepan and cover with 2 inches of cold water. Bring to a boil, reduce the heat, and simmer, covered, for up to 1½ hours, until tender. Use as directed.*

MEDITERRANEAN QUINOA SALAD

Makes 4 servings

¾ cup uncooked quinoa, rinsed well

1½ cups water

pinch salt

1 small English cucumber, diced small

1 cup grape tomatoes, quartered

3 tablespoons diced red onion

8 pitted Kalamata olives, sliced

¼ cup reduced-fat feta cheese crumbles

2 tablespoons chopped fresh mint

1½ tablespoons olive oil

1 tablespoon lemon juice

1. Place the quinoa and water in a medium saucepan with a pinch of salt and bring to a boil.

2. Reduce the heat and simmer over low heat, covered, for 15 minutes, until the quinoa absorbs the water.

3. Remove from the heat and let sit, covered, for 5 minutes, then fluff the quinoa and set aside.

4. Combine the cucumber, tomatoes, red onion, and olives in a large bowl.

5. Add the quinoa, feta, mint, olive oil, and lemon juice; toss to combine.

6. Chill the salad before serving, if desired, or serve warm.

COUSCOUS-STUFFED BAKED TOMATOES

Makes 8 servings

8 large, ripe tomatoes

olive oil, as needed

1 cup whole-wheat couscous, uncooked

2 cups low-sodium vegetable broth, boiling

1 tablespoon canola oil

1 small yellow onion, diced

½ cup diced mushrooms

2 cloves garlic, minced

¼ cup chopped cilantro

2 tablespoons chopped parsley

pinch each salt and pepper

¼ cup whole-wheat breadcrumbs

canola oil cooking spray

1. Preheat the oven to 350°F.

2. Carefully slice the tops off the tomatoes and scoop out and discard the pulp and seeds. Discard the tops, or reserve for another use.

3. Arrange the tomatoes cut side up in a glass baking dish large enough to hold them, and brush the insides with olive oil.

4. Place the couscous in a medium heatproof bowl and pour the boiling broth over it. Stir well, then cover and let sit for 5 minutes before fluffing the couscous with a fork.

5. Heat the canola oil in a medium skillet over medium-high heat. Add the onion, mushrooms, and garlic, then cook for 5 minutes, until the liquid from the mushrooms has cooked off.

6. Stir the onion mixture into the couscous along with the cilantro and parsley, then season with a pinch each of salt and pepper.

7. Spoon the couscous mixture into the tomatoes and sprinkle with breadcrumbs.

8. Spray the tops lightly with cooking spray, then bake for 16 to 18 minutes, until the tomatoes are tender, and serve hot.

SPINACH MOZZARELLA PANINI

Makes 4 servings

8 slices whole-wheat bread

2 to 3 tablespoons olive oil

2 cups baby spinach, packed

4 ounces fresh part-skim mozzarella, sliced thin

salt and pepper

1. Preheat a panini press according to the manufacturer's instructions.

2. Brush one side of each slice of bread with olive oil.

3. Divide half of the spinach among half of the slices of bread, and top the un-oiled side of each with slices of fresh mozzarella. Sprinkle with a pinch each of salt and pepper.

5. Top with the remaining spinach and slices of bread.

6. Grill the sandwiches using the panini press, following the manufacturer's instructions.

7. Cut the sandwiches in half, and serve hot.

BALSAMIC STRAWBERRY AND SPINACH SALAD

Makes 4 servings

6 cups baby spinach, packed

1 cup sliced mushrooms

½ small red onion, sliced thin

1¼ cups diced fresh strawberries, divided

⅓ cup sliced almonds

3 tablespoons olive oil

2 tablespoons balsamic vinegar

pinch dry mustard powder

pinch each salt and pepper

1. Combine the spinach, mushrooms, and red onion in a salad bowl and then divide among 4 salad plates.

2. Divide 1 cup of the diced strawberries among the salads, and top each with 1 to 2 tablespoons sliced almonds.

3. Place the remaining ¼ cup strawberries in a food processor with the olive oil, balsamic vinegar, mustard powder, and a pinch each of salt and pepper.

4. Process until smooth and well combined, then drizzle over the salads. Serve immediately.

ROSEMARY CHICKPEA SOUP

Makes 6 to 8 (1-cup) servings

1 pound dry chickpeas, picked over

1 tablespoon olive oil

2 large yellow onions, coarsely chopped

1 tablespoon minced garlic

8 cups low-sodium chicken broth

2 tablespoons chopped fresh rosemary

1 bay leaf

pinch each salt and pepper

1. Place the chickpeas in a bowl and cover with water by 1 inch. Let soak overnight, then drain.

2. Heat the oil in a large stockpot over medium heat. Add the onions and cook for 10 to 12 minutes, until softened.

3. Stir in the garlic and cook for 2 minutes, then add the chickpeas, chicken broth, rosemary, and bay leaf.

4. Bring the mixture to a boil, then reduce the heat and simmer, covered, for 35 to 40 minutes, until the chickpeas are tender.

5. Remove the bay leaf and season with a pinch each of salt and pepper. Serve hot.

ROASTED TOMATO BASIL BISQUE

Makes 6 (1-cup) servings

2½ pounds ripe Roma tomatoes, halved

1 large yellow onion, sliced

3 tablespoons olive oil, divided

pinch each salt and pepper

1 large carrot, peeled and chopped

1 large stalk celery, chopped

2 tablespoons minced garlic

4 cups low-sodium chicken broth

1 (14.5-ounce) can diced tomatoes

1 bay leaf

1 teaspoon chopped fresh thyme

1 teaspoon chopped fresh oregano

1 cup canned light coconut milk

¼ cup chopped fresh basil

1. Preheat the oven to 400°F. Line a rimmed baking sheet with foil.

2. Toss the Roma tomatoes and onions with 2 tablespoons of the olive oil in a large bowl, then spread them on the baking sheet and season with a pinch each of salt and pepper.

3. Roast the tomatoes and onions for 25 minutes; stir and roast for another 20 to 25 minutes, until lightly charred.

4. Heat the remaining tablespoon of olive oil in a stockpot over medium heat.

5. Stir in the carrots and celery and cook for 4 to 6 minutes.

6. Add the garlic and cook for another 2 minutes before stirring in the chicken broth, canned tomatoes and their juice, bay leaf, thyme, and oregano.

7. Stir in the roasted tomatoes and onions and bring to a boil.

8. Reduce the heat and simmer for 35 minutes, uncovered, then remove from the heat and let cool for 10 minutes.

9. Remove the bay leaf, then puree the soup using an immersion blender.

10. Place the stockpot back over medium heat and whisk in the coconut milk and basil.

11. Adjust the seasonings to taste, and serve hot.

———— ● ● ● ● ————

MEXICAN BLACK BEAN SOUP

Makes 6 to 8 (1-cup) servings

1 tablespoon olive oil

1 large yellow onion, chopped

1 tablespoon minced garlic

1 medium red bell pepper, cored and chopped

1 medium green bell pepper, cored and chopped

1 tablespoon ground cumin

½ to 1 teaspoon cayenne pepper

8 cups low-sodium chicken broth

2 (15-ounce) cans black beans, rinsed and drained

pinch each salt and pepper (optional)

fat-free sour cream, to serve

cilantro sprigs, to serve

1. Heat the oil in a large saucepan over medium heat. Stir in the onion, garlic, and bell peppers. Cook for 6 to 8 minutes, until the onion is translucent and the peppers are tender. Add the cumin and cayenne; stir well.

2. Stir in the chicken broth and black beans, then bring the mixture to a boil.

3. Reduce the heat and simmer for 15 minutes, until the beans are tender.

4. Remove the saucepan from the heat and puree the soup, using an immersion blender, then season with a pinch each of salt and pepper, if desired.

5. Spoon the soup into bowls and serve hot, garnished with a dollop of fat-free sour cream and a sprig of fresh cilantro.

PEAR AND BUTTERNUT SQUASH SOUP

Makes 6 to 8 (1-cup) servings

1 tablespoon olive oil

1 large yellow onion, coarsely chopped

2 medium, ripe pears, peeled, cored, and diced

2 pounds butternut squash, peeled, seeded, and chopped

4 cups water

1 teaspoon grated fresh ginger

pinch each salt and pepper

⅓ cup plain fat-free yogurt

chopped chives, to serve

1. Heat the oil in a stockpot over medium-high heat. Stir in the onion and cook for 5 to 6 minutes, until it is translucent.

2. Add the pears, butternut squash, and water, then add the ginger and a pinch each of salt and pepper.

3. Bring the mixture to a boil, reduce the heat, and simmer for 22 to 25 minutes, until the squash is very tender.

4. Remove the soup from the heat and puree it using an immersion blender. Whisk in the yogurt and adjust the seasonings to taste.

5 . Spoon the soup into bowls and garnish with chopped chives.

CREAMY WALDORF SALAD

Makes 6 to 8 (1-cup) servings

⅓ cup chopped walnuts

2 large apples, cored and sliced thin

1½ cups thinly sliced celery

⅔ cup seedless raisins

⅓ cup plain fat-free yogurt

1½ teaspoons lemon juice

1 teaspoon honey

chopped romaine lettuce, to serve

1. Preheat the oven to 350°F and spread the walnuts on a rimmed baking sheet.

2. Bake for 12 to 15 minutes, stirring occasionally, until lightly toasted, then set aside to cool.

3. Combine the apple, celery, raisins, and walnuts in a medium bowl.

4. In a small bowl, whisk together the yogurt, lemon juice, and honey until smooth.

5. Toss the dressing with the apple mixture until evenly coated.

6. Serve the salad over beds of chopped romaine.

TOMATO, MOZZARELLA, AND PESTO PANINI

Makes 8 servings

16 slices whole-wheat bread

1 cup basil pesto

1 pound fresh part-skim mozzarella, sliced thin

2 large beefsteak tomatoes, sliced thin

salt and pepper

1. Preheat a panini press according to the manufacturer's instructions.

2. Spread about 1 tablespoon of pesto on each slice of bread. Top half with slices of mozzarella and tomato, then season with a pinch each of salt and pepper. Top half with slices of bread.

3. Grill the sandwiches on the panini press according to the manufacturer's instructions.

4. Cut the sandwiches in half and serve hot.

To make your own pesto: *Combine 4 cups fresh basil leaves, ⅓ cup raw pine nuts, and 2 cloves garlic in a food processor. Process until smooth, then pulse in ½ cup grated Parmesan cheese and a pinch of salt. With the processor running, drizzle in up to ½ cup olive oil until you achieve the desired consistency. Yields 1 cup.*

CHICKEN, AVOCADO, MANGO, AND QUINOA SALAD

Makes 4 servings

½ cup quinoa, rinsed well

1 cup water

2 tablespoons olive oil

1 teaspoon minced garlic

1 pound boneless skinless chicken breast, chopped

1 large, ripe avocado, pitted and chopped

1 large, ripe mango, peeled, pitted, and chopped

juice of 2 limes

¼ cup chopped cilantro

1½ tablespoons fresh orange juice

1 tablespoon olive oil

2 teaspoons honey

salt and pepper

1. Combine the quinoa and water in a medium saucepan with a pinch of salt.

2. Bring to a boil, reduce the heat, and simmer, covered, for about 15 minutes, until the quinoa is tender.

3. Remove from the heat and rest for 5 minutes, then fluff the quinoa with a fork.

4. Heat the oil in a large skillet over medium heat. Add the garlic and chicken, stirring to coat with oil. Cook for 6 to 8 minutes, stirring as needed, until the chicken is cooked through.

6. Transfer the quinoa to a large bowl and add the cooked chicken along with the avocado and mango. Toss to combine.

7. Combine the lime juice, cilantro, orange juice, olive oil, honey, and a pinch each of salt and pepper in a small bowl, whisking until smooth and well combined.

8. Toss the salad with the dressing and serve warm.

SALSA-STUFFED BAKED ZUCCHINI

Makes 4 (½-stuffed-zucchini) servings

2 medium zucchini

olive oil, as needed

2 cups diced ripe tomatoes

1 small green bell pepper, cored and diced

½ small red onion, diced

¼ cup chopped cilantro

½ teaspoon ground cumin

pinch each salt and pepper

½ cup whole-wheat breadcrumbs

1. Preheat the oven to 375°F.

2. Trim the ends from the zucchini and cut the zucchini in half lengthwise.

3. Scoop out the flesh from the middle of each zucchini half, leaving a ¼-inch border, and brush the zucchini with olive oil.

4. Chop the zucchini flesh, place in a medium bowl, and stir in the tomatoes, green pepper, red onion, and cilantro.

5. Stir in the cumin and season with a pinch each of salt and pepper.

6. Spoon the tomato mixture into the zucchini halves and arrange them in a baking dish.

7. Sprinkle each zucchini half with breadcrumbs, then bake, uncovered, for 35 to 40 minutes, until the zucchini are tender. Serve hot.

EASY FENNEL APPLE SOUP

Makes 4 to 6 (1-cup) servings

1 tablespoon olive oil

1 large sweet onion, chopped

1 large bulb fennel, and diced

4 cups low-sodium vegetable broth

1 cup water

½ teaspoon chopped fresh tarragon

¼ teaspoon ground ginger

pinch each salt and pepper

3 large Granny Smith apples, cored and diced

toasted sunflower seeds, to serve

ground saffron, to serve

1. Heat the oil in a large saucepan over medium heat.

2. Add the onion and fennel, tossing to coat with oil, then cook for 7 to 9 minutes, until the onion starts to caramelize.

3. Whisk in the vegetable broth, water, ginger, and tarragon, then season with a pinch each of salt and pepper.

4. Stir in the apples and bring to a boil over high heat.

5. Reduce the heat and simmer for 35 minutes, until the ingredients are very tender.

6. Remove from the heat and puree the soup with an immersion blender until smooth.

7. Ladle the soup into bowls and garnish with toasted sunflower seeds and a pinch of ground saffron.

GRILLED PORTOBELLO MUSHROOM BURGERS

Makes 4 servings

¼ cup fat-free mayonnaise

½ cup basil pesto

½ teaspoon grated fresh horseradish

olive oil, as needed

4 whole-wheat burger buns, cut in half

4 large portobello mushroom caps, cleaned well

salt and pepper

⅔ cup reduced-fat blue cheese crumbles

2 cups arugula, rinsed well

1. Whisk together the mayonnaise, pesto, and horseradish in a small bowl; set aside.

2. Preheat a grill to medium-high heat and brush the grates with olive oil.

3. Grill the burger buns until toasted. Spread the pesto mayonnaise onto the buns and set aside.

4. Remove the stems from the mushroom caps, then brush with oil and season with a pinch each of salt and pepper.

5. Place the mushroom caps on the grill, gill side down, and grill for 3 to 4 minutes.

6. Turn the mushrooms over and grill for another 4 to 5 minutes, until tender.

7. Place one grilled mushroom cap on each sandwich bun and top with blue cheese and arugula. Serve hot.

CREAM OF MUSHROOM SOUP

Makes 6 to 8 (1-cup) servings

2 tablespoons olive oil

2 pounds crimini mushrooms, sliced

1 tablespoon minced garlic

1 cup sliced shallots

pinch each salt and pepper

1 teaspoon chopped fresh tarragon

½ cup canned light coconut milk

1. Heat the oil in a large stockpot over medium-high heat.

2. Add the mushrooms, stirring to coat with oil, then cook for 6 to 8 minutes, until most of the water from the mushrooms has cooked off.

3. Set aside 1 cup of the cooked mushrooms, leaving the rest in the stockpot.

4. Add the garlic and shallots to the stockpot, stirring well, then cook for 30 to 60 seconds.

5. Season with a pinch each of salt and pepper, then bring the mixture to a boil.

6. Stir in the tarragon, reduce the heat, and simmer for 5 minutes. Remove from the heat.

7. Puree the soup using an immersion blender, then whisk in the coconut milk.

8. Adjust the seasoning to taste and serve hot, garnished with the reserved mushrooms.

WHOLE-WHEAT PASTA SALAD WITH ARUGULA

Makes 6 to 8 (1-cup) servings

4 cups whole-wheat rigatoni pasta

1 cup plain fat-free yogurt

¼ cup chopped walnuts

¼ cup grated reduced-fat Parmesan cheese

1 teaspoon minced garlic

3 cups arugula, rinsed well, divided

pinch each salt and pepper

½ cup sun-dried tomatoes packed in oil, drained and chopped, to serve

1. Bring a pot of salted water to a boil and add the whole-wheat pasta.

2. Cook the pasta al dente according to the directions on the box—9 to 11 minutes.

3. Drain the pasta and rinse with cold water. Set aside.

4. Combine the yogurt, walnuts, cheese, and garlic in a food processor and process until smooth.

5. Add half the arugula and pulse to blend, then season with a pinch each of salt and pepper.

6. Transfer the cooked pasta to a large bowl and toss with the dressing and the remaining arugula.

7. Chill until ready to serve. Garnish with sun-dried tomatoes before serving.

SWEET POTATO AND CARROT
SOUP WITH GINGER

Makes 4 to 6 (1-cup) servings

1 tablespoon olive oil

¾ cup sliced shallots

2 large sweet potatoes, peeled and diced

2 cups baby carrots, chopped

1-inch piece fresh ginger, peeled and grated

2¼ teaspoons curry powder

4 cups low-sodium chicken broth

pinch each salt and pepper

fat-free sour cream, to serve

1. Heat the oil in a large saucepan over medium-high heat. Stir in the shallots and cook for 2 to 3 minutes, until tender.

2. Add the sweet potato, carrots, and ginger, then stir in the curry powder and cook for 2 minutes more.

3. Whisk in the chicken broth, and bring the mixture to a boil. Reduce the heat and simmer for 20 to 25 minutes, until the vegetables are very tender.

4. Remove from the heat and puree the soup, using an immersion blender. Season with a pinch each of salt and pepper, then serve hot, garnished with a dollop of fat-free sour cream.

SALMON SALAD–STUFFED PITA POCKETS

Makes 4 servings

2 (7-ounce) cans Alaskan salmon in water, drained

3 tablespoons fat-free sour cream

1½ tablespoons fat-free mayonnaise

1 tablespoon lemon juice

1 tablespoon chopped fresh dill

pinch each salt and pepper

2 whole-wheat pitas

1 to 2 cups shredded lettuce

1 medium tomato, sliced thin

½ small English cucumber, sliced thin

1. Flake the salmon into a medium bowl and toss with the sour cream, mayonnaise, and lemon juice. Add the dill and season with a pinch each of salt and pepper.

2. Cut the pitas in half and open them to form pockets. Divide the lettuce, tomato, and cucumber among the pita halves.

3. Stuff each pita pocket with salmon salad and serve immediately.

APPLE ALMOND CHICKEN SALAD

Makes 4 (1-cup) servings

12 ounces boneless, skinless chicken breast, cooked and chopped

½ cup diced celery

¼ cup diced red onion

pinch each salt and pepper

½ cup plain fat-free yogurt

¼ cup reduced-fat mayonnaise

1 teaspoon Dijon mustard

½ teaspoon honey

2 medium apples, cored and diced

chopped lettuce, to serve

3 tablespoons sliced almonds, to serve

1. Combine the chicken, celery, and red onion in a medium bowl and season with a pinch of salt and pepper.

2. In a small bowl, whisk together the yogurt, mayonnaise, mustard, and honey until smooth.

3. Toss the chicken mixture with the dressing.

4. Fold in the diced apples, then chill for 2 to 4 hours before serving.

5. Spoon the chicken salad over a bed of chopped lettuce and sprinkle with almonds to serve.

CHAPTER 8

DINNER RECIPES

---◆◆◆◆---

SPINACH AND RICOTTA WHOLE-WHEAT LASAGNA

Makes 8 to 10 (1-cup) servings

8 ounces whole-wheat lasagna noodles

1 tablespoon olive oil

1 pound lean ground turkey

10 ounces mushrooms, sliced

1 (16-ounce) package frozen spinach, thawed and squeezed dry

2 (14.5-ounce) cans crushed tomatoes

¼ cup chopped fresh basil

pinch each salt and pepper

2 cups part-skim ricotta cheese

2 cups part-skim shredded mozzarella cheese

1. Preheat the oven to 350°F. Lightly grease an 8 x 10-inch glass baking dish.

2. Bring a large pot of salted water to a boil and add the noodles.

3. Cook for 2 minutes less than the directions on the package indicate, then drain and rinse with cool water.

4. Heat the oil in a large skillet over medium-high heat.

5. Add the ground turkey and cook for 5 minutes or so, until evenly browned.

6. Stir in the mushrooms and cook for 6 to 8 minutes, until the mushrooms are tender.

7. Add the spinach, stirring well, then remove from the heat.

8. Combine the tomatoes, basil, salt, and pepper in a food processor and process until smooth.

9. Spread about ½ cup of the tomato sauce in the bottom of the baking dish.

10. Top the sauce with a layer of cooked noodles, cutting them as needed to fit.

11. Drop half of the ricotta over the noodles in heaping tablespoons, then spread evenly.

12. Sprinkle half the turkey and mushroom mixture over the ricotta, followed another ½ cup of tomato sauce.

13. Top the sauce with one third of the shredded mozzarella.

14. Repeat the layers (noodles, remaining ricotta, remaining turkey and mushroom mixture, tomato sauce, half the remaining mozzarella, noodles), and end with the remaining mozzarella. Cover the dish with foil.

15. Bake for 1 hour and 10 minutes, until the sauce is hot and bubbling.

16. Remove the foil and bake for another 8 to 10 minutes, until the cheese is browned.

17. Let the lasagna rest for about 10 minutes before cutting to serve.

BAKED EGGPLANT PARMESAN

Makes 4 servings

2 large eggs

1½ cups whole-wheat breadcrumbs

1 teaspoon dried Italian seasoning

1 large eggplant, sliced ¼ inch thick

1 (24-ounce) jar low-sodium tomato sauce (no added sugar)

1½ cups shredded part-skim mozzarella cheese

1. Preheat the oven to 375°F. Line a rimmed baking sheet with parchment.

2. Beat the eggs in a shallow dish. Combine the breadcrumbs and seasoning in another shallow dish.

3. Dip the eggplant slices in the egg, then dredge in the breadcrumb mixture.

4. Spread the eggplant slices on the baking sheet.

5. Bake for 12 minutes, then flip the slices and bake for another 10 to 12 minutes, until browned.

6. Increase the oven temperature to 475°F. Grease an 8 x 10-inch glass baking dish.

7. Spread one third of the tomato sauce in the baking dish and top with a layer of baked eggplant slices.

8. Sprinkle with one third of the cheese, then repeat the layers, ending with the cheese.

9. Bake for 12 to 15 minutes, until the sauce is bubbling and the cheese is melted. Turn on the broiler.

10. Place the baking dish under the broiler for 2 to 3 minutes, until the cheese is browned.

11. Let cool for 10 minutes before serving.

GREEK-STYLE STUFFED BELL PEPPERS

Makes 6 servings

6 medium red bell peppers

1 tablespoon olive oil

1 medium yellow onion, chopped

1 small zucchini, peeled and diced

2 (14.5-ounce) cans low-sodium stewed tomatoes

1 (10-ounce) package frozen spinach, thawed and squeezed dry

1 teaspoon minced garlic

¼ cup sliced Kalamata olives

2 tablespoons chopped parsley

½ teaspoon dried oregano

½ cup reduced-fat feta cheese crumbles

¼ cup chopped fresh mint, to serve

1. Preheat the oven to 350°F.

2. Slice the tops off the peppers and remove the seeds and membranes.

3. Arrange the peppers in a rectangular glass baking dish.

4. Heat the oil in a large skillet over medium-high heat.

5. Add the onion and cook for 5 to 6 minutes, until translucent.

6. Stir in the zucchini and cook for 3 minutes, until tender.

7. Add the tomatoes, spinach, and garlic; cook for 2 minutes.

8. Remove from the heat and stir in the olives, parsley, and oregano.

9. Spoon the mixture into the peppers and cover the dish with foil.

10. Bake for 30 minutes, then uncover the dish and bake for another 10 minutes.

11. Sprinkle the peppers with feta cheese and bake for 10 to 12 minutes more, until the peppers are tender and the filling is hot.

12. Garnish with the chopped mint and serve.

HERB-CRUSTED PORK TENDERLOIN

Makes 8 to 10 (3-slice) servings

2½ tablespoons olive oil

1½ tablespoons minced garlic

2 teaspoons chopped fresh thyme

1 teaspoon chopped fresh rosemary

1 teaspoon chopped fresh oregano

1 teaspoon dried basil

¼ teaspoon ground cardamom

pinch ground saffron

pinch each salt and pepper

4½ to 5 pounds boneless pork loin

2 large yellow onions, sliced

1. Preheat the oven to 475°F.

2. Combine the olive oil, garlic, thyme, rosemary, oregano, basil, cardamom, saffron, salt, and pepper in a small bowl. Use a fork to mash the mixture into a paste.

3. Rub the herb mixture by hand into the pork tenderloin on all sides.

4. Place the tenderloin fat side down in a roasting pan.

5. Sprinkle the onions around the tenderloin, then roast for 30 minutes.

6. Reduce the oven temperature to 425°F and roast for 55 to 65 minutes more, until the internal temperature reaches 155°F.

7. Remove the tenderloin to a cutting board and cover loosely with a tent of foil.

8. Let rest for 15 minutes before slicing to serve.

GRILLED SALMON WITH MANGO CILANTRO PUREE

Serves 6   Serving size: 1 4-ounce fillet with 2 tablespoons sauce

2 medium, ripe mangos, peeled, pitted, and chopped

1 cup chopped cilantro

1 cup canned light coconut milk

1 clove garlic, minced

2 tablespoons lime juice

1½ pounds boneless salmon fillet, skin on

olive oil, as needed

salt and pepper

1. Combine the mango, cilantro, and coconut milk in a food processor.

2. Process until smooth and well combined, then pulse in the garlic and lime juice.

3. Transfer the puree to a small saucepan and simmer over low heat, covered, while you prepare the salmon.

4. Slice the salmon into 4-ounce fillets, and brush both sides with olive oil.

5. Preheat a grill to high heat and brush the grates with olive oil when hot.

6. Season the salmon with a pinch each of salt and pepper, then place the fillets on the grill, skin side up.

7. Close the grill and cook for 1 to 2 minutes, until grill marks appear.

8. Turn the fillets over and grill skin side down for another 2 to 4 minutes, until the salmon is cooked to the desired doneness.

9. Serve the fillets hot, drizzled with the mango cilantro puree.

ROSEMARY ROASTED CHICKEN WITH VEGETABLES

Serves 6 to 8   Serving size: 2 drumsticks or thighs with 1 cup vegetables

canola oil cooking spray

1 tablespoon olive oil

1 medium yellow onion, coarsely chopped

1 tablespoon minced garlic

3½ to 4 pounds chicken drumsticks and thighs

pinch each salt and pepper

2 cups chopped broccoli florets

1 cup chopped carrots

1 large sweet potato, peeled and chopped

1 red bell pepper, cored and chopped

¼ cup plus 2 tablespoons low-sodium chicken broth, divided

2 tablespoons chopped fresh rosemary

½ teaspoon dried oregano

¼ teaspoon dried thyme

1. Preheat the oven to 400°F. Lightly grease a 9 x 13-inch glass baking dish with cooking spray.

2. Heat the oil in a large skillet over medium-high heat. Add the onion and garlic and cook for 5 to 6 minutes, until the onion is tender.

3. Season the chicken with a pinch of salt and pepper and add to the skillet. Cook the chicken for 2 to 3 minutes on each side, until just browned.

4. Combine the broccoli, carrots, sweet potato, and bell pepper in a medium bowl. Toss with ¼ cup of the chicken broth and the rosemary, oregano, and thyme.

5. Spread the vegetables in the baking dish and top with the chicken and the onion mixture.

6. Drizzle with the remaining 2 tablespoons broth, then roast for 30 minutes.

7. Turn the chicken and stir the vegetables, then roast for another 25 to 30 minutes, until the chicken juices run clear.

8. Let cool for 5 minutes before serving the chicken hot with the vegetables.

BLUE CHEESE TURKEY BURGERS

Makes 6 servings

1¼ pounds lean ground turkey

½ cup whole-wheat breadcrumbs

¼ cup diced red onion

¼ cup reduced-fat blue cheese crumbles

1 tablespoon whole-grain mustard

1 clove garlic, minced

pinch each salt and pepper

6 whole-wheat burger buns, toasted

1. Preheat the broiler in your oven to high heat.

2. Combine the turkey, breadcrumbs, onion, and blue cheese in a large bowl.

3. Stir in the mustard and garlic, then season with a pinch each of salt and pepper.

4. Shape the mixture into 6 even-sized patties by hand, making them about ½ inch thick.

5. Broil the turkey burgers for 4 to 5 minutes on each side, until cooked through.

6. Serve the burgers hot on the toasted buns with your favorite DASH diet–friendly burger toppings.

Suggested Toppings: *sliced tomato, shredded romaine lettuce, sliced red onion*

CHICKEN WITH PASTA PUTTANESCA

Makes 6 to 8 (1½-cup) servings

10 ounces whole-wheat spaghetti

¾ cup assorted pitted olives

6 whole anchovy fillets

1 tablespoon minced garlic

2 tablespoons olive oil

1 medium red onion, sliced thin

2 cups grape tomatoes, halved

1 cup low-sodium chicken broth

2 pounds boneless skinless chicken breast halves

pinch each salt and pepper

½ cup shredded reduced-fat Parmesan cheese

1. Bring a large stockpot of salted water to a boil and add the spaghetti. Cook the spaghetti al dente according to the directions on the package, 9 to 11 minutes. Drain the pasta and set aside.

2. Combine the olives, anchovies, and garlic in a food processor, and pulse until finely chopped.

3. Heat the oil in a large skillet over medium-high heat. Add the red onion and cook for 10 to 12 minutes, until caramelized.

4. Stir in the tomatoes and cook for 3 to 4 minutes, until tender. Add the chicken broth and cook for 2 minutes, then stir in the olive mixture.

5. Push the ingredients in the skillet to the side, add the chicken breast halves, and season with a pinch each of salt and pepper.

6. Cook for 1 to 2 minutes until the underside is browned then flip the chicken breast halves and cook for another 1 to 2 minutes until browned.

7. Reduce the heat to low and cover the skillet—cook for 8 to 10 minutes until the chicken is cooked through. Remove the

chicken breast halves to a cutting board and slice them, then add the chicken back to the skillet.

8. Add the pasta and Parmesan cheese, and toss to combine. Cook until heated through. Serve hot.

COCONUT-CRUSTED BAKED TILAPIA FILLETS

Makes 4 servings

4 (6-ounce) boneless tilapia fillets
salt and pepper
½ cup unsweetened shredded coconut
½ cup whole-wheat breadcrumbs
2 tablespoons coconut flour
½ teaspoon garlic powder
pinch ground cumin
pinch each salt and pepper
2 large egg whites, beaten
lemon wedges, to serve

1. Preheat the oven to 425°F. Line a rimmed baking sheet with foil.

2. Combine the coconut, breadcrumbs, coconut flour, and garlic powder in a shallow dish.

3. Season the tilapia fillets with cumin and a pinch each of salt and pepper. Beat the egg whites in a shallow bowl, then dip the tilapia fillets in the egg.

4. Dredge the fillets in the coconut mixture, coating both sides, then place the fillets on the baking sheet.

5. Bake for 18 to 22 minutes, until the flesh flakes easily with a fork. Serve the fillets hot with lemon wedges.

SWEET POTATO VEGGIE BURGERS

Makes 8 (1 burger) servings

1 large sweet potato

1 (15-ounce) can chickpeas, rinsed and drained

½ small yellow onion, diced

2 tablespoons tahini

½ teaspoon apple cider vinegar

1 clove garlic, minced

1 teaspoon chili powder

¼ teaspoon ground turmeric

pinch each salt and pepper

½ cup whole-wheat breadcrumbs

1 tablespoon olive oil

8 whole-wheat burger buns, toasted

1. Preheat the oven to 400°F.

2. Pierce the sweet potato several times with a knife or a fork, then bake for 45 to 60 minutes, until tender.

3. Cut the sweet potato in half and scoop the flesh into a large bowl.

4. Add the chickpeas, then mash the mixture using a potato masher.

5. Stir in the onion, tahini, vinegar, garlic, chili powder, turmeric, salt, and pepper until well combined. Place the breadcrumbs in a shallow dish.

6. Shape the mixture into 8 even-sized patties by hand, then dredge in the breadcrumbs.

7. Heat the oil in a large skillet over high heat.

8. Add the patties to the skillet and cook for 1 to 2 minutes on each side, until browned.

9. Transfer the patties to a rimmed baking sheet and bake for 10 to 15 minutes, until heated through.

10. Serve the burgers hot on toasted whole-wheat buns with your favorite burger toppings.

Suggested Toppings: *sliced tomato, shredded romaine lettuce, sliced red onion*

———— ●●●● ————

OVEN-BAKED HADDOCK WITH TOMATO SALSA

Serves 4   Serving size: 1 fillet with ½-cup salsa

2 tablespoons olive oil

1 medium yellow onion, diced

1 teaspoon minced garlic

salt and pepper

4 (6-ounce) boneless haddock fillets

2 ripe medium tomatoes, cored and diced

1 small green bell pepper, cored and diced

¼ cup diced red onion

¼ cup chopped cilantro

½ teaspoon ground cumin

pinch cayenne (optional)

1. Preheat the oven to 350°F. Lightly grease a glass baking dish large enough to hold the haddock in one layer.

2. Heat the oil in a medium skillet over medium-high heat. Add the onion and garlic and cook for 6 to 8 minutes, until tender.

3. Season with a pinch each of salt and pepper and cook for 1 minute more.

4. Sprinkle the haddock fillets with a pinch each of salt and pepper and place them in the baking dish.

5. Top with the onion mixture, then bake for 15 to 18 minutes, until the flesh flakes easily with a fork.

6. Combine the tomatoes, green pepper, red onion, cilantro, cumin, and cayenne (if using) in a medium bowl, stirring well.

7. Serve the haddock fillets hot, topped with the fresh tomato salsa.

GINGER SHRIMP AND VEGETABLE STIR-FRY

Serves 4 to 6   Serving size: 3 ounces shrimp, 1-cup vegetables, ½-cup brown rice

1 cup water

¼ cup low-sodium soy sauce

1 tablespoon rice wine vinegar

1 tablespoon arrowroot powder

1 teaspoon honey

2 tablespoons minced fresh ginger

pinch cayenne

4 tablespoons olive oil, divided

1 large yellow onion, chopped

1½ cups chopped broccoli florets

1½ cups chopped cauliflower florets

1½ cups sliced mushrooms

1½ pounds large shrimp, peeled and deveined

pinch each salt and pepper

6 green onions, cut into 2-inch pieces

steamed brown rice, to serve

1. Whisk together the water, soy sauce, vinegar, arrowroot powder, honey, ginger, and cayenne in a small bowl.

2. Heat 1 tablespoon of the olive oil in a large skillet or wok over medium-high heat. Add the onion and cook for 5 to 6 minutes, until translucent.

3. Transfer the onion to a bowl and reheat the skillet with another tablespoon of oil.

4. Add the broccoli and cauliflower, tossing to coat with oil, and sauté for 6 to 8 minutes, until tender-crisp.

5. Spoon the cauliflower and broccoli into the bowl with the onion and add the mushrooms to the skillet.

6. Cook the mushrooms for 3 to 5 minutes, until they are tender and most of the liquid has cooked off.

7. Spoon the mushrooms into the bowl and reheat the skillet with the remaining 2 tablespoons oil.

8. Add the shrimp to the skillet and season with salt and pepper.

9. Cook the shrimp for 1 to 2 minutes on each side, until just opaque and cooked through. Transfer to a plate to keep warm.

10. Stir the sauce, then pour it into the skillet. Cook for 1 to 2 minutes, until thickened.

11. Return the cooked vegetables and shrimp to the skillet, along with the green onion. Toss to combine.

12. Cook until the mixture is just heated through, then serve hot over steamed brown rice.

WHOLE-WHEAT LEMON ARTICHOKE PASTA
Makes 6 (1½-cup) servings

12 ounces whole-wheat bowtie pasta

2 tablespoons olive oil

1 medium yellow onion, chopped

1 (14-ounce) can artichoke hearts in water, drained and chopped

1½ teaspoons minced garlic

2 tablespoons lemon juice

2 tablespoons chopped parsley

1. Bring a large stockpot full of salted water to a boil and add the pasta. Cook the pasta al dente according to the directions on the package, 9 to 11 minutes. Drain the pasta and set it aside.

2. Heat the oil in a large skillet over medium-high heat. Add the onions and artichoke hearts and cook for 3 to 4 minutes, until lightly browned. Stir in the garlic and cook for 1 minute.

3. Add the cooked pasta, lemon juice, and parsley, mixing until well combined. Cook for 1 to 2 minutes, stirring often, until heated through.

WHOLE-WHEAT MARGHERITA PIZZA

Makes 6 (2-to-3 slice) servings

1 cup warm water

1 teaspoon coconut sugar

1 packet active dry yeast

3 cups whole-wheat pastry flour

1 tablespoon olive oil

1 teaspoon salt

1 to 2 medium, ripe tomatoes, sliced thin

1 pound fresh part-skim mozzarella, sliced thin

½ cup thinly sliced basil leaves

1. Whisk together the water and coconut sugar in the bowl of a stand mixer fitted with a dough hook. Sprinkle the yeast over it.

2. Let the mixture set for 10 minutes, then add the flour, oil, and salt. Mix on low speed for 2 minutes, until the dough just starts to come together.

3. Increase the speed to medium and blend until the dough is smooth and elastic—4 to 5 minutes.

4. Coat the dough ball with oil and place it in a bowl. Cover with plastic and let rise for 1 hour, until doubled in size.

5. Turn the dough out onto a lightly oiled surface and divide into 2 pieces. Form each piece into a ball, then cover with plastic and let rise for another 15 to 20 minutes.

6. Preheat the oven to 525°F. Sprinkle 2 baking sheets with flour and then place one dough ball on each baking sheet. Stretch each ball into a 12-inch circle.

7. Divide the tomato slices between the 2 pizza crusts, leaving a ½-inch border around the edge of each. Top the pizzas with slices of mozzarella cheese, then bake for 12 to 15 minutes, until the cheese is melted and lightly browned.

8. Sprinkle the basil over the pizzas, then slice to serve.

WHOLE-WHEAT PENNE WITH FRESH PESTO

Makes 6 (1½-cup) servings

12 ounces whole-wheat penne pasta

2 cups fresh basil leaves, packed

⅓ cup raw pine nuts

2 ounces reduced-fat Parmesan cheese, grated

4 cloves garlic, minced, divided

½ cup olive oil

pinch each salt and pepper

1 tablespoon canola oil

½ small yellow onion, diced

chopped fresh basil, to serve

1. Bring a large stockpot full of salted water to a boil and add the pasta.

2. Cook the pasta al dente according to the directions on the package, 9 to 11 minutes.

3. Drain the pasta and set it aside.

4. Combine the basil and pine nuts in a food processor and process until well combined.

5. Add the Parmesan cheese and 3 cloves of the garlic, pulsing to combine.

6. Scrape down the sides of the food processor bowl and then, with the processor running, drizzle in the olive oil. Process until creamy.

7. Season the pesto with a pinch each of salt and pepper.

8. Heat the canola oil in a deep skillet over medium-high heat.

9. Add the onion and cook for 5 to 6 minutes, until tender.

10. Stir in the remaining clove of garlic and cook for 1 minute, then add the pasta and pesto. Toss to combine.

11. Cook for 2 to 3 minutes, until heated through. Serve hot, garnished with chopped fresh basil.

BAKED ZUCCHINI AND ONION CASSEROLE

Makes 6 to 8 (1½-cup) servings

1 tablespoon olive oil

1 large yellow onion, chopped

1 tablespoon minced garlic

2 medium zucchini, sliced thin

pinch each salt and pepper

canola oil cooking spray

2 cups shredded reduced-fat mozzarella cheese, divided

½ cup whole-wheat breadcrumbs

canola oil, as needed

1. Heat the olive oil in a large skillet over medium heat.

2. Add the onion and cook for 5 to 6 minutes, until translucent.

3. Stir in the garlic and cook for 1 minute more.

4. Add the zucchini and cook for 10 to 12 minutes, until tender, stirring often.

5. Season with a pinch each of salt and pepper, then remove from the heat.

6. Preheat the oven to 375°F. Lightly grease an 8 x 8-inch square glass baking dish with cooking spray.

7. Spread the zucchini and onion mixture in the baking dish and stir in 1 cup of the shredded cheese.

8. Combine the remaining 1 cup cheese with the breadcrumbs in a small bowl, and sprinkle over the zucchini mixture.

9. Drizzle with canola oil and bake for 10 to 12 minutes, until hot and bubbling. Preheat the broiler.

10. Place the casserole under the broiler for 3 to 4 minutes, until lightly browned.

11. Let the casserole rest for 10 minutes before serving.

ZUCCHINI "PASTA" BOLOGNESE

Makes 6   Serving size: 1-cup zucchini pasta with ½ cup sauce

1¼ pounds lean ground turkey

1 large yellow onion, diced

3 (14.5-ounce) cans low-sodium crushed tomatoes

1 (6-ounce) can low-sodium tomato paste

1 tablespoon minced garlic

1½ teaspoons dried oregano

1 teaspoon dried basil

½ teaspoon dried thyme

1 teaspoon olive oil

6 large zucchini, peeled or spiralized into noodles

salt and pepper

1. Cook the ground turkey in a large skillet over medium-high heat until browned.

2. Drain the fat, then stir in the onions and season with a pinch each of salt and pepper.

3. Cook for 3 to 4 minutes, until the onions are translucent.

4. Stir in the tomatoes, tomato paste, garlic, oregano, basil, and thyme.

5. Bring the mixture to a boil, reduce the heat, and simmer for 30 to 40 minutes.

6. Season the sauce with a pinch each of salt and pepper.

7. Heat the oil in a separate large skillet over medium heat.

8. Add the zucchini "pasta" and sauté for 4 to 6 minutes, until heated through and tender.

9. Serve the zucchini "pasta" hot, topped with the Bolognese sauce.

BLACK BEAN QUINOA BURGERS

Makes 6 (1 burger) servings

1 cup water

½ cup quinoa, rinsed well

1 tablespoon olive oil

1 small yellow onion, diced

1 tablespoon minced garlic

1 (15-ounce) can black beans, rinsed and drained

½ cup old-fashioned oats, uncooked

¼ cup whole-wheat flour

1 large egg, beaten

1½ teaspoons ground cumin

¼ teaspoon ground turmeric

pinch each salt and pepper

6 whole-wheat burger buns, toasted

1. Combine the water and quinoa in a small saucepan.

2. Bring the mixture to a boil, reduce the heat, and simmer, covered, for 12 to 15 minutes, until the quinoa absorbs the water.

3. Remove from the heat and fluff the quinoa with a fork.

4. Heat the oil in a medium skillet over medium heat, and add the onion.

5. Cook for 4 to 5 minutes, until the onion is translucent, then add the garlic and cook for 1 minute more.

6. Transfer the mixture to a large bowl, then stir in the beans. Mash the mixture gently, using a fork or potato masher.

7. Stir in the cooked quinoa, oats, and flour along with the egg, cumin, turmeric, salt, and pepper.

8. Shape the mixture by hand into 6 even-sized patties.

9. Arrange the patties on a rimmed baking sheet, then cover and chill for several hours or overnight.

10. Preheat the oven to 400°F, and place the baking sheet in the oven.

11. Cook for 10 to 12 minutes, then flip the patties and bake for another 10 minutes, until cooked through.

12. Serve the burgers hot on toasted whole-wheat buns with your favorite burger toppings.

   Suggested Toppings: *sliced tomato, shredded romaine lettuce, sliced red onion*

—————●●●●————

CHIPOTLE-LIME GRILLED SHRIMP SKEWERS

Makes 6 servings

⅓ cup lime juice

3 tablespoons chopped cilantro

1½ tablespoons olive oil, plus more for the grill

1 teaspoon minced garlic

1 teaspoon chipotle chili powder

1 teaspoon grated lime zest

1½ pounds large shrimp, peeled and deveined

wooden skewers, soaked in water for 1 hour

1. Whisk together the lime juice, cilantro, olive oil, garlic, chili powder and lime zest in a small bowl.

2. Place the shrimp in a zip-top freezer bag, and pour in the marinade.

3. Shake the bag to coat the shrimp, then let marinate for 30 minutes at room temperature.

4. Preheat a grill to medium-high heat and brush the grates with olive oil.

5. Slide the shrimp onto skewers and place the skewers on the hot grill.

6. Cook for 2 to 3 minutes per side, until the shrimp is just cooked through and opaque. Serve hot.

CHERRY-APPLE ROASTED TURKEY BREAST

Makes 6 (4-ounce) servings

3 cups apple cider

1 cup unsweetened cranberry juice

¼ cup kosher salt

¼ cup pure maple syrup

2 tablespoons grated orange zest

8 cups cold water

4-pound bone-in turkey breast

2 cups unsweetened apple juice

1 cup unsweetened cherry juice

½ cup apple cider vinegar

½ cup honey

canola oil cooking spray

pinch ground cardamom

pinch each salt and pepper

1. Whisk together the apple cider, cranberry juice, kosher salt, maple syrup, and orange zest in a large saucepan.

2. Bring the mixture to a boil, reduce the heat, and simmer for 35 minutes. Place the turkey breast in a large glass dish or bowl.

3. Whisk the cold water into the apple cider mixture, then pour it over the turkey breast. Cover and chill for 4 hours.

4. Whisk together the apple juice, cherry juice, apple cider vinegar, and honey in a medium bowl.

5. Preheat the oven to 350°F.

6. Remove the turkey from the liquid and pat it dry. Place it in a roasting pan, skin side up.

7. Spray the turkey breast with cooking spray, then season with a pinch each of ground cardamom, salt, and pepper.

8. Roast for 1 hour and 30 to 45 minutes, basting with the cherry–apple juice mixture every 15 minutes, until the internal temperature reaches 160°F.

9. Transfer the turkey breast to a cutting board and cover loosely with foil. Let the turkey rest for 10 minutes before carving to serve.

PEPPER-CRUSTED BAKED HALIBUT FILLETS

Makes 6 servings

1½ cups whole-wheat breadcrumbs

1½ tablespoons minced garlic

1 tablespoon freshly ground pepper

1½ teaspoons grated lemon zest

1 tablespoon olive oil

6 (6-ounce) boneless halibut fillets

1 cup dry white wine or cooking sherry

salt

lemon wedges, to serve

1. Preheat the oven to 425°F.

2. Combine the breadcrumbs, garlic, pepper, lemon zest, and ½ teaspoon salt in a small bowl.

3. Heat the oil in a large, oven-safe skillet over medium-high heat.

4. Season the fillets with a pinch of salt, and add them to the skillet. Cook for 2 to 3 minutes on each side, until just seared.

5. Drizzle the wine over the fillets, and spoon the breadcrumb mixture over them.

6. Transfer the skillet to the oven and bake for 5 to 6 minutes, until the flesh flakes easily with a fork.

7. Serve hot with lemon wedges.

WHOLE LEMON AND HERB ROASTED CHICKEN

Makes 3 to 4 servings

4 to 4½-pound roasting chicken

olive oil, as needed

pinch each salt and pepper

4 sprigs fresh rosemary

4 sprigs fresh thyme

6 cloves fresh garlic, peeled

6 lemons, halved or quartered, divided

1 large yellow onion, sliced

1 cup dry white wine

½ cup low-sodium chicken broth

2 tablespoons whole-wheat pastry flour

1. Preheat the oven to 425°F.

2. Remove the giblets from the chicken cavity and rinse the whole chicken with cold water, inside and out.

3. Pat the chicken dry with paper towels, and place it breast side up in a roasting pan.

4. Rub the chicken with olive oil, then season with a pinch of salt and pepper.

5. Place the rosemary, thyme, garlic, and 2 lemon halves in the chicken cavity.

6. Tie the chicken legs together with kitchen string, then tuck the tips of the wings under the chicken.

7. Cut the remaining lemons into quarters and scatter them around the chicken with the onion.

8. Roast the chicken for 1 hour and 15 minutes, then check the internal temperature of the thickest part with a meat thermometer.

9. If the internal temperature has not reached 165°F, let the chicken cook for another 15 minutes or so, until done.

10. Remove the chicken to a cutting board and cover loosely with foil. Remove the lemons and onions and discard.

11. Spoon the cooking juices into a medium saucepan and whisk in the white wine.

12. In a small bowl, whisk together the chicken broth and flour, then whisk the mixture into the saucepan.

13. Bring the mixture to a boil, reduce the heat, and simmer until thickened, about 5 minutes.

14. Carve the chicken and serve hot with the gravy.

———— ● ● ● ● ————

DIJON-CRUSTED PORK CHOPS

Makes 4 servings

2½ tablespoons Dijon mustard

1 teaspoon chopped fresh rosemary

¼ teaspoon ground fresh horseradish

pinch each salt and pepper

1 cup whole-wheat breadcrumbs

1 tablespoon olive oil

4 (6-ounce) bone-in pork chops, 6 ounces each

1. Preheat the oven to 400°F.

2. Whisk together the mustard, rosemary, horseradish, salt, and pepper in a small bowl. Place the breadcrumbs in a shallow dish.

3. Brush the mustard mixture onto the pork chops on both sides, then dredge in the breadcrumbs.

4. Heat the oil in a large, oven-safe skillet over medium-high heat.

5. Add the pork chops to the skillet and cook for 2 to 3 minutes on each side, until browned.

6. Transfer the skillet to the oven and bake for 15 to 20 minutes, until the pork chops are cooked through.

SLOW-COOKER BEEF AND MUSHROOM BOURGUIGNON

Makes 6 to 8 (1½-cup) servings

6 slices low-sodium turkey bacon

3 pounds beef sirloin, cut into cubes

pinch each salt and pepper

2 cups dry red wine, divided

2 large yellow onions, chopped

2 large carrots, peeled and chopped

2 large stalks celery, chopped

1 pound white mushrooms, sliced

1 tablespoon low-sodium tomato paste

1 teaspoon minced garlic

1 large bay leaf

2 sprigs fresh thyme

2 sprigs fresh rosemary

1 cup low-sodium beef broth

1. Cook the bacon in a large, heavy skillet over medium-high heat until crisp. Using a slotted spoon, remove the bacon to paper towels to drain. Chop the bacon when cooled.

2. Season the beef with a pinch each of salt and pepper. Return the skillet to medium-high heat and add the beef. Cook for 1 to 2 minutes on each side, until browned.

3. Transfer the beef to the slow cooker, then pour ¼ cup of the wine into the skillet. Simmer for 2 to 3 minutes, scraping up the browned bits from the bottom of the pan.

4. Pour the wine from the pan into the slow cooker, then stir in the onions, carrots, celery, and mushrooms.

5. Add the tomato paste and garlic, then place the bay leaf and sprigs of thyme and rosemary on top of the ingredients in the slow cooker.

6. Pour in the remaining 1¾ cups wine and the broth, then cover the slow cooker and cook on Low for 6 to 8 hours, until the beef is tender.

7. Discard the bay leaf, thyme, and rosemary, then spoon the mixture into bowls and garnish with chopped bacon to serve.

───── ●●●● ─────

BAKED SWORDFISH WITH TROPICAL FRUIT SALSA

Serves 6   Serving size: 1 fillet with ¼ cup salsa

6 (6-ounce) boneless swordfish steaks

olive oil, as needed

salt and pepper

1 cup diced fresh pineapple

1 cup chopped mango

1 small ripe tomato, cored and diced

¼ cup diced English cucumber

2 tablespoons minced red onion

2 tablespoons minced red bell pepper

2 tablespoons chopped cilantro

1 tablespoon lime juice

lemon wedges, for serving

1. Preheat the oven to 400°F.

2. Brush the swordfish steaks with olive oil and season with a pinch each of salt and pepper.

3. Combine the pineapple, mango, tomato, cucumber, onion, red pepper, cilantro, and lime juice in a medium bowl. Toss to combine, and chill until ready to use.

4. Place the steaks on a rimmed baking sheet and bake for 9 to 11 minutes, until just cooked through.

5. Serve the swordfish hot, topped with the salsa and a lemon wedge.

SRIRACHA GRILLED TOFU AND VEGETABLE SKEWERS

Makes 4 servings

1 (16-ounce) package extra-firm tofu, drained and cut into 1-inch cubes

2 medium zucchini, cut into ½-inch slices

1 large red bell pepper, cored and cut into 1-inch chunks

1 medium red onion, cut into 1-inch chunks

1½ cups whole button mushrooms

½ cup low-sodium soy sauce

¼ cup Sriracha sauce

2 tablespoons toasted (dark) sesame oil

pinch ground ginger

oil, for the grill

wooden skewers, soaked in water for 1 hour

lime wedges, to serve

1. Combine the tofu, zucchini, red pepper, onion, and mushrooms in a large bowl.

2. Whisk together the soy sauce, Sriracha, sesame oil, and ginger in a small bowl, then add to the tofu and vegetables. Toss to coat.

3. Cover and chill for 1 hour in the refrigerator.

4. Preheat a grill to medium-high heat and brush the grates with oil.

5. Slide the tofu and vegetables onto the skewers.

6. Place the skewers on the grill and cook for 2 minutes on each side, or until cooked to the desired doneness.

7. Serve the skewers hot with lime wedges.

SLOW-COOKER CHICKEN CACCIATORE

Makes 8 to 10 (1½-cup) servings

¾ cup whole-wheat pastry flour

1 teaspoon salt

½ teaspoon black pepper

2 tablespoons olive oil

3½ to 4 pounds chicken thighs

1 (14.5-ounce) can diced tomatoes in juice

1 large yellow onion, chopped

12 ounces mushrooms, sliced

2 large carrots, sliced thin

1 medium red bell pepper, cored and chopped

1 teaspoon minced garlic

1 cup low-sodium chicken broth

1 cup dry red wine

1. Combine the flour, salt, and pepper in a shallow dish and dredge the chicken thighs in the mixture.

2. Heat the oil in a large skillet over medium-high heat.

3. Add the chicken and cook for 2 to 3 minutes on each side, until browned.

4. Combine the tomatoes with their juice, onion, mushrooms, carrot, red pepper, and garlic in a slow cooker.

5. Stir in the chicken broth and wine, then place the chicken thighs on top.

6. Cover the slow cooker and cook on high for 4 to 6 hours, until the chicken is cooked through. Serve hot.

TEMPEH TIKKA MASALA

Makes 4 servings

MARINATED TEMPEH:

½ cup water

1 teaspoon plain fat-free yogurt

½ teaspoon garam masala

½ teaspoon chili powder

½ teaspoon paprika

pinch ground saffron

1 cup cubed tempeh

1 teaspoon olive oil

TIKKA MASALA:

1 tablespoon olive oil

1 small yellow onion, chopped

1 teaspoon ground coriander

½ teaspoon garam masala

½ teaspoon ground turmeric

¼ teaspoon paprika

¼ teaspoon ground fenugreek

pinch ground saffron

2 large ripe Roma tomatoes, chopped

1 tablespoon minced garlic

1 tablespoon grated fresh ginger

1 mild green chile, minced

2 tablespoons plain fat-free yogurt

2 to 4 tablespoons fat-free or low-fat milk

½ cup chopped cilantro, to serve

1. To prepare the tempeh: Combine the water, yogurt, garam masala, chili powder, paprika, and saffron in a medium bowl.

2. Toss the tempeh with the marinade until coated.

3. Heat a medium skillet over low heat and add the tempeh with the marinade. Cook for 15 to 18 minutes, until the liquid has been absorbed.

4. Add 1 teaspoon olive oil to the skillet, toss with the tempeh, and cook for 2 to 3 minutes over medium heat, until golden brown. Remove the skillet from the heat and set aside.

5. To prepare the tikka masala: Heat 1 tablespoon olive oil in a separate large skillet over medium heat.

6. Add the onion and cook for 6 to 8 minutes, until translucent. Stir in the coriander, garam masala, turmeric, paprika, fenugreek, and saffron.

7. Stir in the tomatoes, garlic, ginger, and chile, and cook for 15 to 18 minutes on medium-low heat, until the mixture is thick.

8. Add the tempeh and yogurt to the skillet, then thin with milk until it reaches the desired consistency.

9. Simmer the mixture for 2 to 3 minutes. Serve hot, garnished with the chopped cilantro.

ROSEMARY GARLIC CRUSTED LAMB CHOPS

Makes 4 (2-to-3-lamb-chop) servings

1½ tablespoons minced garlic

1 tablespoon chopped fresh rosemary

3 tablespoons olive oil

pinch each salt and pepper

10 to 12 bone-in lamb chops, 2 to 2½ ounces each

1. Preheat the broiler in your oven to high heat.

2. Combine the garlic, rosemary, and olive oil in a food processor. Process the mixture until smooth, then season with salt and pepper.

3. Place the lamb chops on a rimmed baking sheet and spread the garlic mixture liberally over them.

4. Broil for 3 to 4 minutes on each side, until cooked to the desired doneness. Transfer the lamb chops to a plate and let rest for 5 minutes before serving.

CHAPTER 9

SIDE DISHES

● ● ● ●

GINGER SNAP PEAS

Makes 4 to 6 (½-cup) servings

2 teaspoons olive oil

3 small shallots, sliced thin

1-inch piece fresh ginger, peeled and grated

1 clove garlic, minced

1 pound sugar snap peas, ends trimmed

½ cup water

pinch each salt and pepper

1. Heat the oil in a large skillet over medium-high heat.

2. Add the shallots, ginger, and garlic, then sauté for 1 to 2 minutes.

3. Stir in the snap peas and sauté for another 2 minutes or so.

4. Add the water and cook, uncovered, for 2 minutes more, until the peas are tender-crisp.

5. Season with a pinch each of salt and pepper. Serve hot.

AVOCADO BROWN RICE SALAD

Makes 4 servings

1 cup brown rice, uncooked

¼ cup low-sodium soy sauce

¼ cup dry white wine

3 tablespoons water

1½ tablespoons honey

1 large English cucumber, sliced thin

2 medium, ripe avocados, pitted and chopped

1 cup chopped cilantro

4 green onions, sliced thin

2 tablespoons lime juice

1 teaspoon grated lime zest

⅓ cup finely chopped peanuts (optional)

1. Bring 2 cups of water to a boil in a large saucepan, then stir in the rice.

2. Bring to a boil, lower the heat to medium, and cook for 30 minutes, uncovered, until tender.

3. Drain the rice, if needed, then set it aside and allow to cool to room temperature.

4. Whisk together the soy sauce, white wine, water, and honey in a small saucepan.

5. Heat the mixture over medium-high heat until the honey has dissolved, about 2 minutes. Set the sauce aside to cool while you prepare the salad.

6. Combine the cooked rice, cucumber, avocado, and cilantro in a large bowl.

7. Add the green onions, lime juice, lime zest, and cooled sauce. Toss to combine.

8. Transfer to a serving bowl, sprinkle with chopped peanuts, if using, and serve.

MUSHROOM AND KALE BUCKWHEAT SALAD

Makes 4 to 6 (¾-cup) servings

¾ cup buckwheat, uncooked

1 large egg white, whisked well

1 cup plus 2 tablespoons water

pinch each salt and pepper

¼ cup grated reduced-fat Parmesan cheese

1 tablespoon olive oil

6 ounces white mushrooms, sliced

½ small yellow onion, diced

2 cloves garlic, minced

4 cups chopped kale, stems removed

1. Place a medium saucepan over medium heat. Toss the buckwheat with the egg in a small bowl.

2. Add the buckwheat to the saucepan and cook for 3 minutes, stirring often, until the grains are dry.

3. Whisk in the water and a pinch of salt, then bring to a boil.

4. Reduce the heat and simmer, covered, for 15 minutes, until the buckwheat absorbs the water.

5. Remove from the heat, and stir in the Parmesan cheese. Place in a large serving bowl.

6. Heat the oil in a large skillet over medium heat.

7. Add the mushrooms, onion, and garlic and cook for 6 to 8 minutes, until the onion is translucent.

8. Stir in the kale and cook for 2 minutes, until just wilted.

9. Add the mushroom and kale mixture to the cooked buckwheat and toss to combine. Season with a pinch of pepper, and serve hot.

WARM VEGGIE QUINOA SALAD

Makes 8 (½-cup) servings

6 tablespoons olive oil

2 cups water plus 3 tablespoons, divided

¼ cup lemon juice

2 teaspoons minced garlic

1 teaspoon honey

1 cup quinoa, rinsed well

1 tablespoon coconut oil

1 small zucchini, diced small

½ medium yellow onion, diced

1 cup cherry tomatoes, halved

¼ cup chopped parsley

¼ cup chopped cilantro

1 teaspoon chopped fresh rosemary

pinch each salt and pepper

1. Combine the olive oil, 3 tablespoons water, lemon juice, garlic, and honey in a food processor.

2. Process until smooth, then season with salt and pepper.

3. Combine the quinoa and the remaining 2 cups water in a medium saucepan.

4. Bring to a boil, reduce the heat, and simmer, covered, for 15 to 20 minutes, until the quinoa has absorbed the liquid. Fluff the quinoa with a fork and set aside.

5. Heat the coconut oil in a medium skillet over medium-high heat.

6. Add the zucchini, onion, and cherry tomatoes, tossing to coat with oil. Season with a pinch each of salt and pepper.

7. Sauté the vegetables for 6 to 8 minutes, until tender, then transfer them to a large bowl.

8. Add the cooked quinoa along with the parsley, cilantro, rosemary, and prepared dressing. Toss to combine, and serve warm.

GARLIC HERB MILLET

Makes 4 servings

2 tablespoons olive oil, divided

¾ cup millet, uncooked

1 tablespoon minced garlic

1 large yellow onion, chopped

2 small green bell peppers, cored and diced

½ cup chopped parsley

¼ cup chopped cilantro

1 teaspoon chopped fresh rosemary

⅓ cup lemon juice

¼ cup tahini

¼ cup water

1 teaspoon honey

pinch each salt and pepper

1. Heat 1 tablespoon of the oil in a medium saucepan over medium heat.

2. Add the millet and garlic, stirring to coat, then cover with 2 inches of boiling water.

3. Simmer the millet, covered, for 20 minutes, then drain and set aside.

4. Heat the remaining 1 tablespoon oil in a large skillet over medium-high heat.

5. Add the onion and green pepper, and cook for 6 to 8 minutes, until tender.

6. Combine the parsley, cilantro, rosemary, lemon juice, tahini, water, and honey in a food processor and process until smooth.

7. Transfer the millet to a serving bowl and add the cooked vegetables and dressing. Toss to combine.

8. Season with a pinch each of salt and pepper and serve.

RED CABBAGE CARROT SLAW

Makes 6 (½-cup) servings

½ medium head red cabbage, shredded

4 cups shredded carrot

½ cup thinly sliced red onion

½ cup rice vinegar

1 teaspoon honey

1 teaspoon olive oil

pinch each salt and pepper

1. Combine the red cabbage, carrot, and onion in a large bowl.

2. Whisk together the vinegar, honey, olive oil, salt, and pepper in a small bowl until smooth.

3. Toss the salad with the dressing until well coated, then chill until ready to serve.

GRILLED ZUCCHINI SLICES

Makes 6 (4-slice) servings

1 tablespoon olive oil, plus more for the grill

1½ teaspoons balsamic vinegar

½ teaspoon honey

pinch each salt and pepper

3 medium zucchini, cut into ½-inch slices

1. Preheat a grill to medium-high heat, and brush the grates with olive oil.

2. Whisk together the olive oil, balsamic vinegar, honey, salt, and pepper in a large bowl.

3. Add the zucchini and toss until coated. Let marinate for 10 minutes.

4. Place the zucchini slices on the grill and cook for 2 minutes.

5. Turn the slices once grill marks appear, and cook for another 2 minutes or so, until tender. Serve hot.

CILANTRO BROWN RICE

Makes 6 to 8 (½-cup) servings

1 tablespoon olive oil

1 small yellow onion, chopped

1 teaspoon minced garlic

pinch each salt and pepper

1 cup brown rice, uncooked

2 cups low-sodium chicken broth

¼ cup lime juice

1 teaspoon grated lime zest

½ cup chopped cilantro

1. Heat the oil in a large skillet over medium heat.

2. Stir in the onion and garlic, then season with a pinch each of salt and pepper. Cook for 3 to 4 minutes, until the onion is translucent, then stir in the rice.

3. Sauté for 2 to 3 minutes, then whisk in the chicken broth, lime juice, and lime zest.

4. Bring the mixture to a boil, reduce the heat, and simmer, covered, for 35 to 40 minutes, until the rice is tender. Fluff the rice with a fork, then stir in the cilantro and serve hot.

SESAME SAUTÉED KALE

Makes 4 servings

2 bunches fresh kale

2 tablespoons light sesame oil

1 tablespoon minced garlic

2 tablespoons water

pinch each salt and pepper

1 to 2 tablespoons sesame seeds, toasted, to serve

1. Rinse the kale well and pat it dry with paper towels.

2. Trim away the thick stems from the kale, then tear the leaves into 2-inch chunks.

3. Heat the oil in a large saucepan over medium heat.

4. Add the garlic and cook for 1 to 2 minutes, until fragrant.

5. Add the kale and the water, and toss to combine. Cover and cook for 1 minute.

6. Stir, and then cover again and cook for 2 minutes more, until the kale is wilted.

7. Transfer the kale to a serving dish and season with a pinch each of salt and pepper. Sprinkle with sesame seeds and serve.

CAJUN-STYLE SEARED SCALLOPS

Makes 6 (4-to-5-scallops) servings

1 tablespoon chili powder

1 teaspoon paprika

1 teaspoon garlic powder

½ teaspoon cayenne

½ teaspoon onion powder

¼ teaspoon dried oregano

¼ teaspoon dried thyme

pinch pepper

1½ pounds sea scallops, rinsed well

1½ tablespoons olive oil

1. Preheat the oven to 350°F.

2. Combine the chili powder, paprika, garlic powder, cayenne, onion powder, oregano, thyme, and pepper in a medium bowl. Add the scallops and toss until evenly coated.

3. Heat the oil in a large, oven-safe skillet over high heat.

4. Add the scallops and cook for 30 to 60 seconds on each side, until seared.

5. Transfer the skillet to the oven and bake for 4 to 5 minutes, until the scallops are just cooked through. Serve hot.

CUCUMBER RED ONION SALAD

Makes 6 to 8 (1-cup) servings

4 medium English cucumbers, sliced thin

pinch salt

2½ tablespoons rice vinegar

2 tablespoons chopped chives

3 cloves garlic, minced

2 teaspoons minced fresh ginger

4 to 5 tablespoons olive oil

2 medium red onions, sliced thin

1. Arrange the sliced cucumbers in a large colander and sprinkle with a pinch of salt. Let the cucumbers drain for 10 minutes while you prepare the rest of the salad.

2. Whisk together the vinegar, chives, garlic, and ginger in a small bowl. While whisking, drizzle in the olive oil—whisk until smooth and emulsified.

3. Combine the cucumbers and red onion in a salad bowl and toss with the dressing. Chill for at least 30 minutes before serving.

● ● ● ●

LEMON PARMESAN BROCCOLI

Makes 6 (1-cup) servings

6 cups chopped broccoli florets

2 tablespoons olive oil

1 tablespoon minced garlic

1½ teaspoons lemon juice

½ teaspoon grated lemon zest

pinch each salt and pepper

¼ cup shaved reduced-fat Parmesan cheese

1. Pour water into a large saucepan to a depth of 1 inch.

2. Place a steamer insert in the saucepan and add the broccoli.

3. Cover and bring to a boil, then steam the broccoli for 3 to 4 minutes, until tender but still crisp.

4. Drain the broccoli and place it in a large bowl.

5. Heat the oil in a small skillet over medium-high heat.

6. Add the garlic and cook for 2 minutes, until fragrant and lightly browned.

7. Stir in the lemon juice and zest. Add to the broccoli and toss to combine.

8. Season with a pinch each of salt and pepper, then sprinkle with shaved Parmesan. Serve hot.

MAPLE SAUTÉED BRUSSELS SPROUTS

Makes 6 (½-cup) servings

1½ pounds Brussels sprouts

1 tablespoon olive oil

pinch each salt and pepper

2 to 3 tablespoons pure maple syrup

1. Trim the stems from the Brussels sprouts and cut them in half.

2. Pour water into a large saucepan to a depth of 1 inch. Place a steamer insert in the saucepan.

3. Add the Brussels sprouts, then cover and bring to a boil.

4. Steam the Brussels sprouts for 3 to 4 minutes, until tender but still crisp. Remove from the pan.

5. Heat the oil in a medium skillet over medium-high heat.

6. Add the Brussels sprouts, tossing to coat with oil. Sprinkle with a pinch each of salt and pepper.

7. Stir in the maple syrup and sauté for 6 to 8 minutes, until tender. Serve hot.

AMARANTH TABBOULEH SALAD

Makes 4 to 5 (1-cup) servings

½ cup uncooked amaranth, rinsed well

1½ cups water

2 small stalks celery, diced

1 large English cucumber, diced

1 small red onion, diced

1 cup cherry tomatoes, halved

¼ cup chopped parsley

¼ cup chopped fresh mint

2 tablespoons olive oil

grated zest and juice of ½ lemon

pinch each salt and pepper

1. Combine the amaranth and water in a medium saucepan.

2. Bring the mixture to a boil, reduce the heat, and simmer for 20 minutes, until the amaranth absorbs most of the water.

3. Combine the celery, cucumber, onion, tomatoes, parsley, mint, olive oil, lemon juice and zest, salt, and pepper in a large bowl, tossing well to combine.

4. Drain the amaranth and rinse under cold water until cool.

5. Toss the amaranth with the salad mixture and chill until ready to serve.

GARLIC MASHED CAULIFLOWER

Makes 4 (½-cup) servings

1 medium head cauliflower, chopped into florets

¼ cup low-sodium vegetable broth

1 tablespoon fat-free or low-fat milk

2 teaspoons olive oil

1 teaspoon minced garlic

salt and pepper

1. Bring a large saucepan of water to a boil, then add the chopped cauliflower and a pinch of salt.

2. Boil for 8 to 10 minutes, until the cauliflower is very tender.

3. Drain the cauliflower and pat dry with paper towels, then place it in a food processor.

4. Add the vegetable broth, milk, olive oil, and garlic.

5. Process until smooth, then season with a pinch each of salt and pepper. Serve hot.

GARLIC SAUTÉED SPINACH

Makes 4 servings

1 tablespoon olive oil
3 cloves garlic, sliced thin
2 pounds baby spinach
pinch each salt and pepper

1. Heat the oil in a large saucepan over medium heat.

2. Add the garlic and cook for 1 to 2 minutes, until fragrant and lightly browned.

3. Using a slotted spoon, remove the garlic to paper towels to drain.

4. Reheat the skillet over medium heat.

5. Add the spinach, tossing to coat with oil.

6. Cover and cook for 4 to 5 minutes, until the spinach is just wilted.

7. Transfer the spinach to a bowl, then add the garlic and toss to combine.

8. Season with a pinch each of salt and pepper. Serve hot.

PARMESAN WILD RICE PILAF

Makes 4 servings

3 teaspoons olive oil, divided

½ small yellow onion, diced

1 cup wild rice

3 cups low-sodium chicken broth

2 cups sliced crimini mushrooms

pinch each salt and pepper

2 tablespoons dry white wine

¼ cup grated reduced-fat Parmesan cheese

1. Heat 2 teaspoons of the oil in a medium saucepan over medium heat.

2. Stir in the onion and cook for 4 to 5 minutes, until softened.

3. Add the wild rice and cook for 30 seconds, then whisk in the chicken broth.

4. Bring to a boil, reduce the heat, and simmer for 40 to 45 minutes, until tender.

5. Drain the rice and set aside.

6. Heat the remaining teaspoon of oil in a large skillet over medium-high heat.

7. Stir in the mushrooms and season with a pinch each of salt and pepper.

8. Sauté for 6 to 8 minutes, until the mushrooms are tender, then stir in the wine.

9. Cook for 2 minutes, until the liquid has cooked off, then stir in the wild rice and Parmesan cheese. Serve hot.

CHAPTER 10

SNACKS AND DESSERTS

— • • • • —

CREAMY DILL YOGURT DIP WITH VEGGIES

Makes 6 to 8 (¼-cup) servings

1 large English cucumber, peeled

1¾ cups plain fat-free yogurt

¾ cup fat-free sour cream

2 tablespoons lemon juice

1 teaspoon minced garlic

½ teaspoon grated fresh horseradish

2 tablespoons chopped fresh dill

salt and pepper

sliced vegetables, to serve

1. Grate or shred the cucumber, then spread it in a colander and sprinkle with salt. Let the cucumber rest for 30 minutes, then spread it on a clean towel and wring it out, squeezing as much moisture from the cucumber as possible.

2. Combine the yogurt, sour cream, lemon juice, garlic, and horseradish in a medium bowl.

3. Whisk in the dill and season with a pinch each of salt and pepper. Stir in the cucumber, then cover and chill for 2 hours before serving with sliced vegetables.

GREEK-STYLE BRUSCHETTA BITES

Makes 24 (2-bruschetta-slice) servings

1 large whole-grain baguette, sliced ¼ inch thick

canola or olive oil cooking spray

3 ripe Roma tomatoes, cored and diced

1 cup artichoke hearts packed in water, drained and chopped

¼ cup Kalamata olives, pitted and sliced

2 tablespoons chopped parsley

1 teaspoon minced garlic

1 tablespoon olive oil

⅓ cup reduced-fat feta cheese crumbles

2 tablespoons chopped fresh mint

pinch each salt and pepper

1. Preheat the broiler in your oven to high heat.

2. Arrange the baguette slices on a rimmed baking sheet and spray lightly with cooking spray.

3. Broil for 1 to 2 minutes, until just toasted. Set aside.

4. Combine the tomatoes, artichoke hearts, olives, parsley, and garlic in a medium bowl.

5. Add the olive oil and feta and toss to combine, then season with the mint and a pinch each of salt and pepper.

6. Spoon some of the bruschetta mixture onto each toasted baguette slice, and serve immediately.

ROASTED RED PEPPER HUMMUS

Makes 8 to 10 (2-tablespoon) servings

2 medium red bell peppers

1 (15.5-ounce) can chickpeas or 1¾ cups cooked chickpeas, rinsed and drained

1 tablespoon minced garlic

½ teaspoon grated fresh horseradish

¼ cup diced yellow onion

pinch each salt and pepper

3 to 4 tablespoons olive oil

whole-wheat pita chips and sliced vegetables, to serve

1. Preheat the oven to 500°F.

2. Place the peppers on a rimmed baking sheet and roast for 30 to 40 minutes, until charred.

3. Remove from the heat and cover immediately with aluminum foil. Set aside for 30 minutes.

4. Unwrap the peppers when they are cool enough to handle, and slice the tops off.

5. Cut the peppers into quarters and remove the seeds and the charred skin.

6. Chop the peppers and place them in a food processor with the chickpeas, garlic, horseradish, onion, salt, and pepper.

7. Process the mixture until smooth and well combined.

8. With the food processor running, drizzle in the olive oil until the hummus reaches the desired consistency.

9. Spoon the hummus into a bowl and serve with whole-wheat pita chips and sliced vegetables.

CREAMY SPINACH AND ARTICHOKE DIP

Makes 8 (¼-cup) servings

1 (10-ounce) package frozen spinach, thawed

2 cups plain fat-free yogurt

1 (8-ounce) package reduced-fat cream cheese

2 tablespoons trans fat–free margarine

1½ cups grated reduced-fat Parmesan cheese

1 (14-ounce) can artichoke hearts in water, drained and chopped

1½ teaspoons minced garlic

½ teaspoon grated fresh horseradish

pinch each salt and pepper

whole-wheat pita chips, to serve

1. Squeeze as much moisture from the spinach as you can, then set it aside.

2. Combine the yogurt, cream cheese, margarine, and Parmesan cheese in a large saucepan over medium heat.

3. Stir the mixture until it is melted and well combined.

4. Remove from the heat and stir in the artichoke hearts and spinach, along with the garlic and horseradish.

5. Season with a pinch each of salt and pepper and serve warm with whole-wheat pita chips.

ROASTED GARLIC CAULIFLOWER "HUMMUS"

Makes 6 (2-to-3-tablespoon) servings

1 medium head cauliflower, cut into florets

4 or 5 cloves garlic, peeled

⅓ cup tahini

4 tablespoons olive oil, divided

1 to 2 tablespoons fresh lemon juice

salt

1. Preheat the oven to 400°F. Line a rimmed baking sheet with parchment.

2. Toss the cauliflower florets and garlic with up to 2 tablespoons of olive oil in a large bowl, then spread them on the baking sheet.

3. Sprinkle lightly with salt, then roast for 40 minutes, turning halfway through.

4. Let the cauliflower and garlic cool slightly, then transfer to a food processor. Process the mixture until smooth, then pulse in the tahini, 2 tablespoons olive oil, lemon juice, and a pinch of salt.

5. If the mixture seems too thick, add up to a tablespoon of water to thin it to the desired consistency.

CHILI BAKED SWEET POTATO FRIES

Makes 4 servings

6 medium sweet potatoes, peeled

2 tablespoons olive oil

1 tablespoon chili powder

pinch cayenne (optional)

1. Preheat the oven to 450°F. Line a rimmed baking sheet with parchment.

2. Slice the sweet potatoes into thin strips and toss with the oil, chili powder, and cayenne (if using) in a large bowl.

3. Spread the sweet potatoes on the baking sheet in a single layer. Bake for 20 minutes, turning occasionally, until golden brown.

4. Remove from the oven and let the fries cool for 5 to 10 minutes before serving.

WHOLE-GRAIN PUMPKIN WALNUT BREAD

Makes 8 to 10 (1-slice) servings

canola oil cooking spray

1¼ cups whole-wheat pastry flour

½ cup oat bran

¾ teaspoon baking powder

½ teaspoon baking soda

1½ teaspoons ground cinnamon

½ teaspoon ground nutmeg

pinch salt

pinch ground cardamom

⅓ cup coconut sugar

⅓ cup canola oil

⅓ cup fat-free or low-fat milk

¼ cup honey

1 large egg, beaten

1¼ cups pumpkin puree

1½ teaspoons vanilla extract

½ to 1 cup chopped walnuts

1. Preheat the oven to 350°F. Grease a regular loaf pan with cooking spray.

2. Combine the flour, oat bran, baking powder, baking soda, cinnamon, nutmeg, salt, and ground cardamom in a medium bowl.

3. In a separate medium bowl, whisk together the coconut sugar, canola oil, milk, honey, and egg.

4. Whisk in the pumpkin puree and vanilla extract until smooth.

5. Add the dry ingredients to the wet mixture in small batches, stirring until smooth after each addition, then fold in the chopped walnuts.

6. Spread the batter in the prepared pan and bake for 55 to 60 minutes, until a knife inserted in the center comes out clean.

7. Let cool for 15 minutes in the pan, then turn out onto a wire rack to cool completely.

HONEY BANANA OVERNIGHT OATS

Makes 6 servings

1½ teaspoons coconut oil

4 ripe bananas, peeled and sliced

2½ teaspoons vanilla extract

½ teaspoon ground cinnamon

2 to 3 tablespoons honey

3 cups fat-free or low-fat milk

1½ cups steel-cut oats, uncooked

1½ tablespoons ground flaxseed

1. Heat the oil in a medium saucepan over medium heat.

2. Stir in the bananas, vanilla extract, and cinnamon.

3. Cook for 2 to 3 minutes, stirring often, until the bananas are caramelized.

4. Stir in the honey, then remove from the heat and set aside.

5. Combine the milk, oats, and ground flaxseed in a medium bowl.

6. Divide the mixture among 6 half-pint glass jars.

7. Spoon the banana mixture into the jars, dividing it as evenly as possible.

8. Stir the ingredients in the jars, then cover with the lids and refrigerate overnight.

9. Enjoy your oats cold, or warm them in the microwave before serving.

WHOLE-WHEAT BANANA CHOCOLATE CHIP BREAD

Makes 10 to 12 (1-slice) servings

canola oil cooking spray

⅓ cup unsweetened applesauce

¼ cup fat-free or low-fat milk

¼ cup light brown sugar, packed

¼ cup honey

½ tablespoon vanilla extract

2 large eggs, beaten

1¼ cups mashed banana (about 3 medium bananas)

1¾ cups whole-wheat pastry flour

1¼ teaspoons baking soda

1 teaspoon ground cinnamon

pinch ground ginger

¼ teaspoon salt

½ cup reduced-fat mini chocolate chips

1. Preheat the oven to 350°F. Spray a loaf pan with cooking spray.

2. Combine the applesauce, milk, brown sugar, honey, and vanilla extract in a medium bowl, stirring until smooth. Whisk in the eggs, then fold in the banana.

3. In a separate medium bowl, stir together the flour, baking soda, cinnamon, ginger, and salt.

4. Whisk the dry ingredients into the wet mixture in small batches until smooth and well combined.

5. Fold in the chocolate chips, then spread the batter in the prepared pan.

6. Bake for 60 to 65 minutes, until a knife inserted in the center comes out clean.

7. Let the bread cool for 10 minutes in the pan, then turn out onto a wire rack to cool completely.

SPICED CARROT CAKE MUFFINS

Makes 12 servings

1½ cups whole-wheat pastry flour

½ cup light brown sugar, packed

1 tablespoon ground cinnamon

1¼ teaspoons baking powder

¾ teaspoon baking soda

½ teaspoon ground nutmeg

pinch ground cardamom

pinch salt

1½ cups unsweetened applesauce

1 cup grated carrot

¼ cup old-fashioned oats, uncooked

1. Preheat the oven to 350°F. Line 12 cups of a regular muffin pan with paper liners.

2. Combine the flour, brown sugar, cinnamon, baking powder, baking soda, nutmeg, cardamom, and salt in a medium bowl.

3. In a separate medium bowl, stir together the applesauce and grated carrots.

4. Whisk the wet ingredients into the dry mixture in small batches, and stir until just combined.

5. Spoon the batter into the prepared pan, filling the cups about three fourths full.

6. Sprinkle the muffins with the oats, then bake for 22 to 26 minutes, until a knife inserted in the center comes out clean.

7. Let the muffins cool for 5 minutes in the pan, then turn out onto a wire rack to cool completely.

WHOLE-WHEAT ALMOND BUTTER BROWNIES

Makes 16 servings

1 cup whole-wheat pastry flour

⅓ cup unsweetened cocoa powder

1 teaspoon baking powder

½ teaspoon baking soda

pinch salt

1 cup coconut sugar

1¼ cups unsweetened applesauce

1 large egg, beaten

⅓ cup trans fat–free margarine

1 cup reduced-fat semisweet chocolate chips

3 to 4 tablespoons smooth almond butter

1. Preheat the oven to 350°F. Grease an 8 x 8-inch square glass baking dish.

2. Combine the flour, cocoa powder, baking powder, baking soda, and salt in a medium bowl.

3. In a separate medium bowl, beat together the coconut sugar, applesauce, and egg.

4. Combine the margarine and chocolate chips in a double boiler over low heat.

5. Heat the mixture until the chocolate is melted, then whisk smooth.

6. Remove from the heat and whisk the chocolate mixture into the sugar mixture.

7. Whisk in the dry ingredients in small batches until just combined.

8. Spread the batter in the prepared pan.

9. Heat the almond butter in a microwave-safe bowl in 10-second intervals on high heat until melted.

10. Drizzle the melted almond butter over the brownie batter and swirl gently with a butter knife.

11. Bake the brownies for 35 to 42 minutes, until a knife inserted in the center comes out clean.

12. Let the brownies cool in the pan on a wire rack to room temperature before cutting into squares.

————•◆◆•————

ORANGE POMEGRANATE BROWN RICE PUDDING

Makes 6 (½-cup) servings

2 cups water

¾ cup brown rice, uncooked

½ cup fresh orange juice

1 teaspoon grated orange zest

pinch ground cardamom

3½ cups fat-free evaporated milk

3 tablespoons low-fat sweetened condensed milk

¼ cup coconut sugar

3 tablespoons pomegranate seeds

1 ripe orange, peeled and chopped

1. Bring the water to a boil in a medium saucepan.

2. Whisk in the rice, then simmer, covered, for about 20 minutes, until the rice is nearly tender.

3. Remove from the heat, then stir in the orange juice, orange zest, cardamom, evaporated milk, condensed milk, and coconut sugar.

4. Return to medium heat and cook, stirring often, until thick and creamy, about 20 minutes.

5. Remove from the heat and spoon the rice pudding into bowls.

6. Serve topped with the pomegranate seeds and chopped orange.

CHERRY DATE ENERGY BALLS

Makes about 24 (1-ball) servings

2 cups raw cashews

1 cup unsweetened shredded coconut

1 cup pitted Medjool dates

1 cup dried cherries

2 tablespoons coconut oil

1 teaspoon vanilla extract

pinch salt

pinch ground cardamom

1. Line a rimmed baking sheet with parchment. Combine the cashews and coconut in a food processor.

2. Pulse until it forms a crumbled mixture, then add the dates, cherries, coconut oil, vanilla extract, salt, and ground cardamom.

3. Process the mixture until it forms a sticky, doughlike batter.

4. Pinch off pieces of the dough and roll it into balls by hand.

5. Arrange the balls on the baking sheet and freeze for 1 hour, until firm. Store leftover energy balls in an airtight container in the refrigerator or at room temperature.

WHOLE-GRAIN BLUEBERRY ALMOND MUESLI

Makes 8 (½-cup) servings

1½ cups old-fashioned oats, uncooked

1½ cups plain fat-free yogurt

¾ cup fat-free or low-fat milk

pinch salt

1 medium apple, cored and diced

1 cup fresh blueberries

½ cup toasted almonds, chopped

honey, to serve

1. Combine the oats, yogurt, milk, and salt in a medium bowl.

2. Cover the bowl with plastic and chill in the refrigerator for 8 to 12 hours or overnight.

3. Stir in the apple, blueberries, and almonds.

4. Spoon the muesli into bowls and drizzle with honey to serve.

CINNAMON BAKED APPLE CHIPS

Makes 4 servings

4 large sweet apples

ground cinnamon to taste

1. Preheat the oven to 200°F. Line a rimmed baking sheet with parchment.

2. Slice the apples as thinly as possible, using a mandoline or a very sharp knife.

3. Spread the apple slices on the baking sheet in a single layer.

4. Sprinkle with cinnamon, then bake for 1 hour.

5. Carefully flip the apple slices, then bake for another 1½ to 2 hours, until the slices are no longer moist.

6. Turn off the oven and let cool until the apples are crisp.

7. Store in airtight containers at room temperature.

MAPLE RAISIN OATMEAL BAKE

Makes 16 servings

2½ cups fat-free or low-fat milk

¾ cup unsweetened applesauce

3 tablespoons canola oil

2 large eggs, beaten

3 to 4 tablespoons pure maple syrup

1½ teaspoons vanilla extract

2½ cups old-fashioned oats, uncooked

1 cup raisins

1 teaspoon baking powder

½ teaspoon ground nutmeg

pinch salt

1. Preheat the oven to 375°F. Lightly grease an 8 x 10-inch baking dish.

2. Whisk together the milk, applesauce, oil, eggs, maple syrup, and vanilla extract in a large bowl.

3. In a medium bowl, stir together the oats, raisins, baking powder, nutmeg, and salt.

4. Stir the dry ingredients into the wet mixture until smooth and well combined.

5. Spread the mixture evenly in the prepared baking dish.

6. Bake for 20 to 25 minutes, until a knife inserted in the center comes out clean.

7. Let the baked oatmeal cool for 5 minutes or so, then cut into squares to serve.

HONEY BAKED BANANA CHIPS

Makes 4 servings

4 to 5 large bananas, peeled

2 tablespoons fresh lemon juice

1 teaspoon honey

pinch ground cinnamon

1. Preheat the oven to 250°F. Line a rimmed baking sheet with parchment.

2. Slice the bananas as thinly as possible.

3. Whisk together the lemon juice, honey, and cinnamon in a medium bowl, then toss with the banana slices.

4. Arrange the slices in a single layer on the baking sheet.

5. Bake for 90 minutes, then flip the slices and bake for another 30 minutes, until crisp.

6. Let the banana chips cool in the oven with the heat turned off. Store in an airtight container.

VANILLA ALMOND RICE PUDDING

Makes 6 to 8 (½-cup) servings

3 cups fat-free or low-fat milk

1 cup brown rice, uncooked

3 tablespoons honey

1 teaspoon vanilla extract

½ teaspoon almond extract

pinch ground cinnamon

¼ cup sliced almonds

1. Whisk together the milk and rice in a medium saucepan over medium-high heat.

2. Bring the milk to a boil, reduce the heat, and simmer for 30 minutes, covered, until the rice is tender.

3. Remove from the heat and whisk in the honey, vanilla extract, almond extract, and cinnamon.

4. Spoon into bowls and garnish with sliced almonds.

WHOLE-WHEAT CHOCOLATE ZUCCHINI BREAD

Makes 8 to 10 (1-slice) servings

2 cups grated or shredded zucchini

1⅔ cups whole-wheat pastry flour

⅓ cup unsweetened cocoa powder

¾ teaspoon baking powder

¾ teaspoon baking soda

¼ teaspoon salt

⅔ cup coconut sugar

½ cup unsweetened applesauce

¼ cup fat-free or low-fat milk

2 large eggs, beaten

1½ teaspoons vanilla extract

1. Preheat the oven to 350°F. Grease a regular loaf pan.

2. Spread the zucchini on a clean towel, then roll it up and wring out as much moisture as possible.

3. Combine the flour, cocoa powder, baking powder, baking soda, and salt in a medium bowl.

4. In a separate medium bowl, beat together the coconut sugar, applesauce, milk, eggs, and vanilla extract.

5. Stir the dry ingredients into the wet mixture until smooth and well combined, then fold in the zucchini.

6. Spread the batter in the prepared pan and bake for 55 to 60 minutes, until a knife inserted in the center comes out clean.

7. Let cool in the pan for 10 minutes, then turn out onto a wire rack to cool completely.

CHERRY LIME GRANITA

Makes 6 (½-cup) servings

2 cups fresh cherries, pitted

⅔ cup coconut sugar

⅔ cup water

juice of 4 limes

lime wedges, to serve

fresh mint sprigs, to serve

1. Place the cherries in a food processor and process until smooth.

2. Strain the cherry puree through a fine-mesh sieve into a bowl, pressing the mixture down to release as much liquid as possible. Discard the flesh.

3. Combine the coconut sugar and water in a small saucepan over medium-high heat.

4. Bring the mixture to a boil and stir until the sugar is completely dissolved.

5. Remove from the heat and whisk in the lime juice and strained cherry juice.

6. Cover with plastic and chill for several hours, until cold.

7. Spread the mixture in a shallow glass dish and freeze.

8. Stir the mixture after an hour and freeze again—continue stirring once an hour until the granita is frozen but still slightly slushy.

9. Spoon the granita into dessert cups and serve each with a lime wedge and a sprig of mint.

BLUEBERRY ALMOND CRUMBLE

Makes 6 servings

3 cups fresh blueberries, rinsed well

1 tablespoon arrowroot powder

¼ cup plus 2 tablespoons coconut sugar, divided

pinch ground cinnamon

pinch ground ginger

½ cup old-fashioned oats, uncooked

2 tablespoons whole-wheat pastry flour

pinch salt

2 tablespoons coconut oil

¼ cup thinly sliced almonds

1. Preheat the oven to 350°F.

2. In a large bowl, toss the blueberries with the arrowroot powder, 2 tablespoons of the coconut sugar, and a pinch each of cinnamon and ginger.

3. Spread the blueberries in a 9-inch glass pie plate.

4. In a medium bowl, combine the oats, flour, and salt with the remaining ¼ cup coconut sugar.

5. Cut in the coconut oil until it forms a crumbled mixture, then stir in the sliced almonds.

6. Spread the mixture over the berries and bake for 30 to 35 minutes, until the berries are bubbling and the topping is browned.

7. Let the crumble cool for 10 minutes or so, then serve warm.

FLOURLESS CHOCOLATE CAKE

Makes 8 (1-slice) servings

canola oil cooking spray

½ cup reduced-fat semisweet chocolate chips

½ cup trans fat–free margarine

¾ cup coconut sugar

3 large eggs, beaten

½ cup unsweetened cocoa powder, plus more for dusting over top

fresh fruit or sorbet, to serve

1. Preheat the oven to 375°F. Grease an 8-inch round cake pan with cooking spray.

2. Cut a circle of parchment paper the size of the cake pan and use it to line the bottom, then grease the parchment with cooking spray.

3. Combine the chocolate chips and margarine in a double boiler over low heat.

4. Heat the chocolate and margarine until melted, then whisk until smooth.

5. Whisk in the coconut sugar, then beat in the eggs, one at a time, until smooth.

6. Add the cocoa power, a few tablespoons at a time, whisking until smooth after each addition.

7. Spread the batter in the prepared pan and bake for 22 to 25 minutes, until a thin crust forms on the top.

8. Cool the cake on a wire rack in the pan for 5 minutes, then turn out onto a plate to cool completely.

9. Dust the cake with extra cocoa powder, if desired. Serve warm with fresh fruit or sorbet.

CREAMY AVOCADO CHOCOLATE MOUSSE

Makes 6 (½-cup) servings

3 ripe avocados, pitted and chopped

3 tablespoons fat-free or low-fat milk

½ cup unsweetened cocoa powder

⅓ cup honey

1 teaspoon vanilla extract

1. Place the avocado in a food processor and process until smooth.

2. Add the milk, cocoa powder, honey, and vanilla extract.

3. Blend for 30 to 60 seconds, until smooth, then spoon into dessert cups.

4. Chill for 30 minutes before serving.

CINNAMON RAISIN QUINOA BOWLS

Makes 4 (1-cup) servings

1 cup quinoa

2 cups fat-free or low-fat milk, plus more to serve

2 to 3 tablespoons honey or brown sugar

⅓ cup raisins

½ teaspoon ground cinnamon

1. Place the quinoa in a medium bowl and cover with water. Stir by hand, then rinse the quinoa until the water runs clear.

2. Drain the quinoa and set it aside.

3. Pour the milk into a medium saucepan and bring to a boil over medium-high heat.

4. Whisk in the quinoa and return the mixture to a boil.

5. Reduce the heat to medium-low and simmer, covered, for 12 to 15 minutes, until the quinoa has absorbed most of the liquid.

6. Remove the saucepan from the heat and fluff the quinoa with a fork.

7. Stir in the honey or brown sugar along with the raisins and cinnamon, then cover and let rest for 15 minutes.

8. Spoon the quinoa into bowls and serve warm, drizzled with fat-free or low-fat milk, if desired.

———— • • • • ————

CHOCOLATE CHIA SEED PUDDING

Makes 4 servings

1½ cups fat-free or low-fat milk

¼ cup plus 1 tablespoon chia seeds

¼ cup unsweetened cocoa powder

3 to 4 tablespoons honey

fresh fruit, to serve

1. Combine the milk, chia seeds, and cocoa powder in a food processor or blender.

2. Blend on high speed until smooth and well combined.

3. Transfer to a medium bowl, and whisk in the honey to taste.

4. Cover with plastic and chill for at least 3 to 6 hours or overnight, until thick.

5. Transfer the mixture back to the food processor or blender and blend until smooth.

6. Spoon into bowls and serve with fresh fruit.

OATMEAL WALNUT COOKIES

Makes about 4 dozen (1-cookie) servings

2 cups old-fashioned oats, uncooked

1 cup whole-wheat pastry flour

¾ teaspoon baking soda

1 teaspoon ground cinnamon

pinch salt

½ cup tahini

¼ cup trans fat–free margarine, at room temperature

1½ cups coconut sugar

1 large egg plus 1 egg white, beaten

1 teaspoon vanilla extract

½ cup chopped walnuts

1. Preheat the oven to 350°F. Line 2 baking sheets with parchment.

2. Combine the oats, flour, baking soda, cinnamon, and salt in a medium bowl.

3. In a separate large bowl, beat together the tahini and margarine until smooth.

4. Beat in the coconut sugar until well combined, then whisk in the egg, egg white, and vanilla extract.

5. Stir the flour and oat mixture into the sugar mixture until just combined, then fold in the walnuts.

6. Pinch off pieces of cookie dough and roll them into 1-inch balls.

7. Place the balls on the prepared baking sheets, spacing them about 2 inches apart, and flatten gently by hand.

8. Bake for 14 to 16 minutes, rotating the pans halfway through, until the edges are just browned.

9. Let cool for 2 to 3 minutes on the pans, then transfer to a wire rack to cool completely.

BALSAMIC POACHED PEARS
WITH BLACKBERRIES

Makes 4 servings

4 large, ripe pears

2 cups dry red wine

1 cup water

1 teaspoon ground cinnamon

pinch ground cardamom

½ teaspoon vanilla extract

1 cup balsamic vinegar

⅓ cup coconut sugar

fresh blackberries, to serve

1. Leaving the stems intact, peel the pears and scoop out the cores from the bottom.

2. Whisk together the wine, water, cinnamon, cardamom, and vanilla extract in a medium saucepan over medium heat.

3. Bring the mixture to a simmer, then add the pears to the liquid.

4. Simmer for 30 minutes, until the pears are tender, then remove the pears from the liquid with a slotted spoon.

5. Whisk together the balsamic vinegar and coconut sugar in a small saucepan.

6. Bring the mixture to a boil over high heat, reduce the heat, and simmer for 12 to 15 minutes, until thick and syrupy.

7. Divide the pears among 4 bowls, then drizzle with the balsamic glaze and top with fresh blackberries to serve.

SLOW-COOKER CINNAMON APPLESAUCE

Makes 10 to 12 (½-cup) servings

6 pounds apples (your choice)

1 cup organic apple cider or apple juice, unsweetened

juice of 1 lemon

½ cup coconut sugar

1 to 2 teaspoons ground cinnamon

1. Peel and core the apples, then cut them into slices and place in a slow cooker.

2. Stir in the apple cider, lemon juice, coconut sugar, and cinnamon.

3. Cover the slow cooker and cook on Low for 7 to 8 hours or overnight, until the apples are very tender.

4. Turn off the slow cooker and puree the apples using an immersion blender or blend them in batches using a food processor.

5. Spoon the applesauce into jars and let cool to room temperature before covering with lids and storing in the refrigerator.

MAPLE CRANBERRY BAKED APPLES

Makes 6 servings

6 apples, unpeeled (your choice)

⅓ cup unsweetened dried cranberries

¼ cup unsweetened shredded coconut

1 tablespoon pure maple syrup

¼ teaspoon ground cinnamon

⅔ cup unsweetened apple juice

1. Slice the tops off the apples and carefully cut out the cores. Arrange the apples in a microwave-safe glass dish.

2. Stir together the cranberries, coconut, maple syrup, and cinnamon in a small bowl. Spoon the cranberry mixture into the apples, then pour the apple juice over them.

3. Cover the dish with plastic, and microwave on High for 6 to 8 minutes, until the apples are tender. Let the apples cool for 5 minutes before serving.

CONCLUSION

Think back to the beginning of this book and try to recall your answers to these four questions:

Do you frequently experience gas, bloating, or indigestion?

Do you suffer from chronic fatigue or muscle aches?

Do you struggle to maintain a healthy weight, or are you trying to lose weight?

Do you have trouble falling asleep at night or concentrating during the day?

Now that you understand more about toxins and the dangers of unhealthy eating habits, your answers to those questions might be what you need to push yourself to make true and lasting changes to your lifestyle. Do not jump headfirst into the DASH diet thinking that it will solve all of your problems, but recognize this program for what it is—a tool to help you make healthy changes to your lifestyle and your diet in order to cleanse your body of harmful toxins and to reduce your risk for heart disease. The DASH diet detox program is not intended to be a magical cure-all, but its principles are firmly rooted in wholesome nutritional practices that have the potential to transform your health and your body.

Switching to a new diet is never easy, and especially in this case, it is not something you should rush. Follow the tips and tricks provided in this book to ease into the DASH diet in order to minimize your withdrawal symptoms and to ensure that you get started on the right foot. If you are not ready to commit to a full four weeks (28 days) on the DASH diet detox program, that is perfectly fine—give the 14-day program a try instead. If, however, you have taken the information in this book to heart and have come to understand that the DASH diet is a practical tool for long-term health and wellness, consider making a commitment to try the program for a full 28 days.

No matter which program you choose, the 14-day or 28-day version, it will take only a few days before you start to see and feel the benefits of the DASH diet detox program. Your body will start to feel lighter, and you may experience relief from digestive issues such as gas, bloating, and diarrhea. A few days more and you will find that your concentration and cognitive performance have improved—you may no longer feel fatigued and cloudy. Many people who commit to the full 28-day DASH diet detox program also experience weight loss or relief from symptoms associated with various chronic diseases. Just remember that you are an individual, so your body may respond to the DASH diet detox program differently than someone else's might. Be patient with yourself and give the program time to do its job. If you are able to commit to the program for its full duration, you will find that, at the end, you feel like a completely new person. In fact, it is my hope that you will have decided that the DASH diet is a program you can follow for the rest of your life.

If you are ready to take back control of your health and make some positive changes to your lifestyle and dietary habits, commit yourself to either the 14-day or the 28-day DASH diet detox program and get started!

APPENDIX

Glossary of Important Terms

Basal metabolic rate (BMR)—The number of calories your body needs on a daily basis to maintain basic metabolic functions such as respiration and digestion.

Biotoxins—Toxins with a biological origin. Examples include neurotoxins, hemotoxin, and necrotoxin.

Chronic disease—A long-lasting condition that can be controlled but not cured. Examples include Alzheimer's disease, asthma, diabetes, cancer, and heart disease.

Detox—To stop taking unhealthy or harmful foods, drinks, and other substances into your body for a period of time, in order to improve your health.

Environmental toxins—Toxins to which you may be exposed through air, water, and land. Examples include cleaning products, pesticides, and pollution.

Fad diet—A diet or eating pattern that promotes short-term weight loss, generally with no regard for long-term maintenance.

Heart disease—A range of conditions affecting the heart, including coronary artery disease, stroke, high blood pressure, cardiac arrest, congestive heart failure, and arrhythmia.

Hypertension—Abnormally high blood pressure.

Internal toxins—Toxins that are created inside the human body. Examples include chronic viral infections, chronic stress, anxiety, and negative thinking.

Lifestyle disease—A disease associated with the way a person lives. Examples include heart disease, obesity, stroke, and type 2 diabetes.

Lifestyle toxins—Toxins to which you are exposed due to lifestyle choices. Examples include tobacco, processed foods, prescription drugs, and refined sugars.

Refined grains—Grains that have been milled to remove the bran and germ; this process gives the product a longer shelf life and finer texture, but removes dietary fiber and other nutrients.

Toxins—Poisonous manmade compounds, or those occurring in nature or found in the body in the form of microorganisms that have an adverse impact on immune function

Whole foods—Foods that have been refined or processed as little as possible and are free from additives and other artificial substances.

Whole grains—Grains or products made with whole, unprocessed grains.

Withdrawal—Physical and mental symptoms that occur after stopping or reducing your intake of a certain substance.

Low-Calorie DASH Diet Snacks

"Because it has an emphasis on real foods, heavy on fruits and vegetables, balanced with the right amount of protein, DASH is the perfect weight loss solution. It is filling and satisfying. Because it is healthy, you can follow it for your whole life."

—The DASH Diet Eating Plan, DashDiet.org

Both the 14-day and the 28-day DASH diet detox meal plans are designed to make your transition into the diet as smooth and simple as possible. By providing you with a list of meals to prepare each day, the DASH diet detox plan takes some of the weight off your shoulders—you do not have to stress about what you will be eating each day. Going in to the DASH diet detox program, you need to determine what your goals are and then take steps to ensure that you reach those goals. If your hope is to lose weight while following the DASH diet detox, stick to the meal plans provided, including the serving suggestions, to keep from overeating. If you simply want to improve your health and nutrition, follow the programs as they are but feel free to add an extra snack or two throughout the day if you need something to tide you over from one meal to the next. Here is a list of low-calorie snacks that are approved for the DASH diet:

- 1 small banana
- 2 to 3 cups air-popped popcorn
- 1 small orange
- ½ cup plain fat-free Greek yogurt
- 1 small apple
- 1 large handful shelled pistachios
- 1 fresh kiwifruit
- 1 cup chopped watermelon
- 1 cup ripe cherries
- 1 cup fresh blackberries

- 1 brown rice cake
- 6 to 8 whole-wheat crackers
- 2 tablespoons hummus, 6 baby carrots
- ½ cup fresh fruit salad
- 2 fresh apricots
- 1 small box of raisins
- ½ cup strawberries, 2 tablespoons fat-free yogurt
- 1 large tomato, 1 tablespoon grated reduced-fat Parmesan
- ½ cup fat-free yogurt, 1 teaspoon honey
- 6 ounces apple cider with cinnamon
- 2 cups fresh raspberries
- 1 cup blueberries
- 3 small squares dark chocolate
- ⅓ cup rolled oats, ¼ cup fresh berries
- Small baked sweet potato
- Apple with 2 teaspoons peanut butter
- 1 cup fresh mango
- 1 whole-grain waffle, ¼ cup berries
- 1 cup seedless grapes
- 1 apple baked with 1 teaspoon brown sugar
- 3 clementines
- 1 cup unsweetened applesauce
- 1 handful toasted almonds
- 1 small scoop fat-free frozen yogurt
- ½ whole-wheat English muffin with 1 tablespoon jam

Bonus DASH Diet Smoothies

"The best smoothies are made with natural, all real, nutrient-dense ingredients that provide vitamins and oils necessary for good, more complete nutrition. . . . Drinking a smoothie in the morning keeps you from indulging in empty carbohydrates like donuts and removes the temptation of the drive-through. In fact, a smoothie made [the right] way packs more usable nutrition than most multivitamins."

—Health Benefits of Smoothies, The Science of Eating[19]

Although subsisting on a diet of only fresh juices and smoothies is not recommended, as mentioned at the beginning of this book, fresh fruit and vegetable smoothies do provide some important benefits that can help you to achieve your goals when following the DASH diet. Fresh smoothies made from fruits and vegetables—often referred to as "green" smoothies—are a great way to boost your consumption of fresh produce without having to scarf down a giant salad or a plate full of fruit. Smoothies can be made with a wide variety of different ingredients in all kinds of flavor combinations. Depending on the ingredients you use, green smoothies can be incredibly indulgent, tasting more like dessert than a healthy snack.[13]

In addition to being a great way to increase your consumption of fruits and vegetables, green smoothies can be a good way to keep your daily calorie count low if you are trying to lose weight on the DASH diet detox program. By substituting a fresh smoothie made from low-calorie fruits and vegetables for your typical high-calorie meal, you can shave a couple hundred calories off your daily intake. If you do this a few times a week, you could lose 1 pound per week (or more). It is important to remember that green smoothies should be used as a tool to support other healthy eating habits—you should not make smoothies the only food you eat during the day, because doing so could cause you to consume too few calories, and you might miss out on important nutrients that come from other foods.

If you are interested in giving green smoothies a try, choose a few of your favorite fruits and vegetables and just throw them into a blender with some water or fruit juice. If you prefer to take a more structured approach, give one of the delicious recipes included in this appendix a try. Once you find a few smoothies you like, feel free to incorporate them into your DASH diet detox meal plan, swapping them for one of your meals or snacks a few times per week.

KIWI GREEN APPLE SMOOTHIE

Serves 1

2 kiwifruit, peeled and sliced

1 small green apple, cored and diced

1 cup plain fat-free yogurt

½ cup ice cubes

¼ cup unsweetened apple juice

1. Combine all of the ingredients in a high-speed blender. Blend on high speed for 30 to 60 seconds, until smooth.

2. Pour the smoothie into a large glass and serve immediately.

DECADENT PEANUT BUTTER BANANA SMOOTHIE

Serves 1

1 large frozen banana, peeled and sliced

2 tablespoons smooth peanut butter

1½ cups fat-free or low-fat milk

½ cup plain fat-free yogurt

pinch ground cinnamon

1. Combine the banana and peanut butter in a high-speed blender. Add the milk, yogurt, and cinnamon, then blend until smooth.

2. Pour the smoothie into a large glass and serve immediately.

TROPICAL PINEAPPLE KIWI SMOOTHIE

Serves 2

1½ cups frozen chopped pineapple

1 kiwifruit, peeled and sliced

1 cup fresh orange juice

½ cup plain fat-free yogurt

½ cup ice cubes

¼ cup shredded unsweetened coconut

1. Combine the pineapple, kiwi, and orange juice in a blender. Blend the ingredients for 30 to 60 seconds on high speed, until smooth. Add the yogurt, ice, and coconut, then blend until smooth.

2. Pour the smoothie into 2 large glasses and serve immediately.

BERRY, BEET, AND APPLE SMOOTHIE

Serves 1

1½ cups frozen blueberries

1 small beet, peeled and chopped

1 cup unsweetened apple juice

1 cup plain fat-free yogurt

1 tablespoon chia seeds

1 teaspoon grated fresh ginger

1. Combine the blueberries, beet, and apple juice in a high-speed blender. Blend for 30 to 45 seconds, until smooth. Add the yogurt, chia seeds, and ginger, then blend until smooth.

2. Pour the smoothie into a large glass and serve immediately.

TRIPLE BERRY SUPREME SMOOTHIE

Serves 2

1 cup frozen strawberries

½ cup frozen blueberries

½ cup frozen blackberries

1 cup plain fat-free yogurt

½ cup fresh orange juice

¼ cup ice cubes

¼ cup chopped fresh mint

1. Place the strawberries, blueberries, and blackberries in a high-speed blender. Add the yogurt, orange juice, ice cubes, and mint, then blend until smooth.

2. Pour the smoothie into 2 large glasses and serve immediately.

CARROT, APPLE, AND GINGER SMOOTHIE

Serves 2

2 cups baby spinach, packed

1 tablespoon chopped fresh ginger

1 cup unsweetened apple juice

1 medium apple, cored and chopped

1 medium carrot, peeled and diced

½ cup ice cubes

1 teaspoon honey (optional)

1. Combine the spinach, ginger, and apple juice in a high-speed blender. Blend until smooth, then add the apple, carrot, ice cubes, and honey (if using) and blend until smooth.

2. Pour into 2 large glasses and serve immediately.

COOLING CUCUMBER MELON SMOOTHIE

Serves 1

1 cup chopped kale, stems removed

¼ cup fresh mint leaves

1 cup unsweetened apple juice

1 cup chopped honeydew melon

½ small English cucumber, peeled and diced

½ cup ice cubes

1. Combine the kale, mint, and apple juice in a high-speed blender. Blend for 30 to 45 seconds, until smooth. Add the honeydew, cucumber, ice, and peppermint, and blend until smooth.

2. Pour the smoothie into a large glass and serve immediately.

AVOCADO WALNUT GREEN SMOOTHIE

Serves 1

½ ripe avocado, pitted and chopped

1 small frozen banana, peeled and chopped

1 cup coconut water

½ cup ice cubes

2 tablespoons chopped walnuts

1 tablespoon lime juice

1. Combine the avocado, banana, and coconut water in a high-speed blender. Blend for 30 to 60 seconds, until smooth. Add the ice cubes, walnuts, and lime juice, and blend until smooth.

2. Pour the smoothie into a large glass and serve immediately.

SIMPLE STRAWBERRY BANANA SMOOTHIE

Serves 1

1 cup frozen strawberries

1 medium frozen banana, peeled and sliced

½ cup fat-free or low-fat milk

1 cup ice cubes

½ cup plain fat-free yogurt

pinch ground cinnamon

pinch ground cardamom

1. Combine the strawberries, banana, and milk in a high-speed blender. Blend until well combined, then add the ice cubes, yogurt, cinnamon, and cardamom. Blend the mixture for 30 to 60 seconds, until smooth.

2. Pour the smoothie into a large glass and serve immediately.

CELERY GREEN APPLE SMOOTHIE

Serves 1

1 large stalk celery, chopped

1 small green apple, cored and chopped

½ small seedless cucumber, peeled and diced

1 cup ice cubes

½ cup unsweetened apple juice

½ cup water

1. Combine all ingredients in a high-speed blender and blend for 30 to 60 seconds.

2. Pour the smoothie into a large glass and serve immediately.

BOUNTIFUL BLUEBERRY MINT SMOOTHIE

Serves 1

1¼ cups frozen blueberries

1 small frozen banana, peeled and sliced

½ cup fresh orange juice

½ cup water

¼ cup chopped fresh mint

1 teaspoon lemon juice

1. Combine the blueberries and banana in a blender with the orange juice and water. Blend until smooth, then add the mint and lemon juice. Blend the mixture on high speed for 30 to 60 seconds, until smooth.

2. Pour the smoothie into a large glass and serve immediately.

CUCUMBER, KALE, AND BANANA SMOOTHIE

Serves 1

1 cup chopped kale, stems removed

½ small English cucumber, peeled and sliced

½ cup fat-free or low-fat milk

1 small frozen banana, peeled and sliced

½ cup plain fat-free yogurt

1 teaspoon raw honey

1. Place the kale and cucumber in a blender with the milk and blend until smooth. Add the banana, yogurt, and honey, then blend until smooth and well combined.

2. Pour the smoothie into a large glass and serve immediately.

CREAMY CHERRY YOGURT SMOOTHIE

Serves 1

1 cup frozen pitted cherries

½ cup frozen strawberries

½ cup fresh orange juice

1 cup plain fat-free yogurt

1 tablespoon chia seeds

1. Combine the cherries, strawberries, and orange juice in a high-speed blender. Blend for 30 to 45 seconds, until smooth.

2. Add the yogurt and chia seeds and blend until smooth, then pour into a large glass and serve immediately.

BEAUTIFUL BROCCOLI KALE SMOOTHIE

Serves 2

2 cups frozen broccoli florets

1 cup chopped kale, stems removed

1 cup unsweetened apple juice

1 large frozen banana, peeled and sliced

1 teaspoon honey

½ teaspoon chopped fresh rosemary

1. Place the broccoli, kale, and apple juice in a blender. Blend until smooth, then add the banana, honey, and rosemary.

2. Blend until smooth, then pour into a large glass and serve immediately.

——————•◆◆◆•——————

MERRY PEACH MANGO SMOOTHIE

Serves 2

1 cup fresh or frozen chopped mango

1 cup fresh or frozen sliced peaches

1 small fresh or frozen banana, peeled and sliced

½ cup fresh orange juice

1 cup plain fat-free yogurt

½ cup ice cubes

1. Combine the mango, peaches, and banana in a high-speed blender. Add the orange juice and blend until smooth. Add the yogurt and ice cubes, then blend until smooth.

2. Pour the smoothie into 2 large glasses and serve immediately.

——————•◆◆◆•——————

CELERY, CUCUMBER, AND LIME SMOOTHIE

Serves 1

2 large stalks celery, sliced

½ small English cucumber, peeled and diced

½ cup coconut water

½ cup ice cubes

2 tablespoons lime juice

2 tablespoons chopped fresh mint

1. Combine the celery, cucumber, and coconut water in a high-speed blender. Blend for 30 to 45 seconds, until smooth.

2. Add the ice cubes, lime juice, and mint, and blend until smooth. Pour into a large glass and serve immediately.

GLOWING GREEN GRAPE SMOOTHIE

Serves 1

1 cup seedless green grapes

1 cup baby spinach, packed

½ cup unsweetened apple juice

½ cup ice cubes

¼ cup plain fat-free yogurt

1. Combine the grapes, spinach, and apple juice in a blender. Blend on high speed for 30 to 45 seconds, until smooth and well combined. Add the ice cubes and yogurt, and blend until smooth.

2. Pour the smoothie into a large glass and serve immediately.

ROCKIN' RASPBERRY BANANA SMOOTHIE

Serves 1

1 cup frozen raspberries

½ frozen banana, peeled and sliced

½ cup fat-free or low-fat milk

½ cup plain fat-free yogurt

1 teaspoon lemon juice

1. Place the raspberries and banana in a blender. Add the milk, yogurt, and lemon juice, then blend until smooth.

2. Pour the smoothie into a large glass and serve immediately.

SASSY STRAWBERRY KIWI SMOOTHIE

Serves 1

1 cup frozen sliced strawberries

1 cup baby spinach, packed

1 kiwifruit, peeled and sliced

1 cup coconut water

½ cup ice cubes

1 teaspoon honey

1. Combine the strawberries, spinach, and kiwi in a high-speed blender. Blend on high speed for 30 seconds, then add the coconut water, ice cubes, and honey.

2. Blend until smooth and well combined. Pour the smoothie into a large glass and serve immediately.

SPINACH, MANGO, AND BANANA SMOOTHIE

Serves 1

2 cups baby spinach, packed

1 cup fat-free or low-fat milk

1 small frozen banana, peeled and sliced

½ cup frozen chopped mango

1 tablespoon ground flaxseed

1. Combine the spinach and milk in a blender. Blend until smooth, then add the banana, mango, and flaxseed and blend for 60 seconds.

2. Pour the smoothie into a large glass and serve immediately.

MARVELOUS MANGO GINGER SMOOTHIE

Serves 1

1 cup frozen chopped mango

½ cup plain fat-free yogurt

1 cup ice cubes

¼ cup fresh orange juice

1 teaspoon grated fresh ginger

1. Combine the mango and yogurt in a high-speed blender. Blend for 30 seconds, until smooth, then add the ice, orange juice, and ginger. Blend until smooth and well combined.

2. Pour the smoothie into a large glass and serve immediately.

CHOCOLATE COCO-BANANA SMOOTHIE

Serves 1

1 large frozen banana, peeled and sliced

½ cup fat-free or low-fat milk

½ cup canned light coconut milk

4 to 5 ice cubes

2 tablespoons unsweetened shredded coconut

1 tablespoon unsweetened cocoa powder

pinch ground cinnamon

1. Combine the banana, milk, and coconut milk in a high-speed blender. Blend until smooth, then add the ice cubes, coconut, cocoa powder, and cinnamon. Blend for 30 to 60 seconds, until smooth and well combined.

2. Pour the smoothie into a large glass and serve immediately.

PUMPKIN PIE SMOOTHIE

Serves 1

½ cup pumpkin puree

½ cup fat-free or low-fat milk

½ cup ice cubes

pinch ground cinnamon

pinch ground nutmeg

pinch ground ginger

1 tablespoon honey (optional)

1. Combine the pumpkin puree and milk in a blender. Blend on high speed until smooth, then add the ice cubes, cinnamon, nutmeg, ginger, and honey (if using). Blend for 30 to 60 seconds, until smooth and well combined.

2. Pour the smoothie into a large glass and serve immediately.

GLORIOUS GARDEN GREENS SMOOTHIE

Serves 1

1½ cups baby spinach, packed

1 cup chopped kale, stems removed

1 cup unsweetened apple juice

2 tablespoons chopped fresh basil

2 tablespoons chopped parsley

1 tablespoon chopped fresh mint

1 teaspoon honey

1. Combine the spinach, kale, and apple juice in a blender and blend until smooth. Add the basil, parsley, mint, and honey, then blend for 30 to 45 seconds.

2. Pour the smoothie into a large glass and serve immediately.

DREAMY ORANGE CREAM SMOOTHIE

Serves 1

1 small frozen banana, peeled and sliced thin

½ ripe orange, peeled and divided into sections

½ cup plain fat-free yogurt

¼ cup fresh orange juice

1 teaspoon grated orange zest

1. Combine the banana, orange, and yogurt in a blender. Blend until smooth, then add the orange juice and zest. Blend until smooth.

2. Pour the smoothie into a large glass and serve immediately.

STRAWBERRY, SPINACH, AND KALE SMOOTHIE

Serves 1

1 cup baby spinach, packed

1 cup chopped kale, stems removed

1 cup unsweetened apple juice

1 cup frozen strawberries

½ small frozen banana, peeled and chopped

1 teaspoon wheatgrass powder

1. Combine the spinach, kale, and apple juice in a high-speed blender. Blend for 30 to 60 seconds, until smooth, then add the strawberries, banana, and wheatgrass powder.

2. Blend until smooth and well combined. Pour the smoothie into a large glass and serve immediately.

WACKY WATERMELON SMOOTHIE

Serves 1

1½ cups chopped watermelon

½ cup frozen strawberries

½ cup plain fat-free yogurt

3 to 4 ice cubes

2 tablespoons fresh orange juice

1 teaspoon honey

1. Combine the watermelon, strawberries, and yogurt in a high-speed blender. Add the ice cubes, orange juice, and honey. Blend the mixture until smooth.

2. Pour the smoothie into a large glass and serve immediately.

PEACHY PEAR AND PINEAPPLE SMOOTHIE

Serves 1

1 cup frozen sliced peaches

½ cup frozen chopped pineapple

½ pear, cored, peeled, and chopped

1 cup fat-free or low-fat milk

¼ cup plain fat-free yogurt

1. Place the peaches, pineapple, and pear in a blender. Add the milk and yogurt, then blend on high speed until smooth.

2. Pour the smoothie into a large glass and serve immediately.

SPINACH, AVOCADO, AND LIME SMOOTHIE

Serves 1

2 cups baby spinach, packed

½ ripe avocado, pitted and chopped

1 cup unsweetened apple juice

½ cup ice cubes

2 tablespoons lime juice

1 teaspoon grated lime zest

1. Combine the spinach, avocado, and apple juice in a blender. Blend on high speed for 30 to 45 seconds, until smooth. Add the ice cubes, lime juice, and zest, then blend until smooth.

2. Pour the smoothie into a large glass and serve immediately.

BLACKBERRY BANANA SMOOTHIE

Serves 1

1½ cups frozen blackberries

1 small frozen banana, peeled and sliced

½ cup fresh orange juice

½ cup plain fat-free yogurt

2 to 3 drops vanilla extract

1. Place the blackberries, banana, and orange juice in a blender. Blend until smooth and then add the yogurt and vanilla extract. Blend until smooth.

2. Pour the smoothie into a large glass and serve immediately.

End Notes

1. "Your Guide to Lowering Blood Pressure." U.S. Department of Health and Human Services. http://www.nhlbi.nih.gov/files/docs/public/heart/hbp_low.pdf
2. "DASH Diet: Healthy Eating to Lower Your Blood Pressure." Mayo Clinic: Nutrition and Healthy Eating. http://www.mayoclinic.org/healthy-living/nutrition-and-healthy-eating/in-depth/dash-diet/art-20048456?pg=2
3. "In Brief: Your Guide to Lowering Your Blood Pressure with DASH." U.S. Department of Health and Human Services. NIH Publication No. 06-5834. December 2006. http://www.nhlbi.nih.gov/files/docs/public/heart/dash_brief.pdf
4. "DASH Diet and High Blood Pressure." WebMD. http://www.webmd.com/hypertension-high-blood-pressure/guide/dash-diet?page=1
5. Gonzalez, Kelly. "Calorie Know-How: Get the Equation Right to Get Results!" BodyBuilding.com. http://www.bodybuilding.com/fun/calorie-know-how-get-equation-right-to-get-results.htm
6. Blumenthal, Brett. "10 Worst Food Additives and Where They Lurk." Gaiam Life. http://life.gaiam.com/article/10-worst-food-additives-where-they-lurk
7. "Toxins and the Immune System." Your Immune System. http://immunedisorders.homestead.com/toxins.html
8. Ewers, Keesha. "What Are Toxins, Where Do Toxins Come From?" Natural Choice Network. http://www.naturalchoice.net/blogs/Art11_Toxins.html#.VQG9JfzF9DQ
9. Hyman, Mark. "Is There Toxic Waste in Your Body?" Dr.Hyman.com. http://drhyman.com/blog/2010/05/19/is-there-toxic-waste-in-your-body-2/#close
10. Aragon, Britta. "7 Signs You May Have Too Many Toxins in Your Life." Mind Body Green. http://www.mindbodygreen.com/0-13737/7-signs-you-have-too-many-toxins-in-your-life.html
11. "12 Benefits of Detoxing the Body." Bembu.com. http://bembu.com/detox-benefits
12. "Lowdown on Sodium." DASH Diet Oregon. http://www.dashdietoregon.org/why/The-Lowdown-on-Sodium
13. "Sodium Health Risks and Disease." Harvard School of Public Health. http://www.hsph.harvard.edu/nutritionsource/salt-and-sodium/sodium-health-risks-and-disease/
14. "To Protect Your Heart, Your Sodium to Potassium Ratio Is More Important Than Your Overall Salt Intake." Mercola.com. http://articles.mercola.com/sites/articles/archive/2014/08/25/sodium-potassium-ratio.aspx
15. Blumenthal, James A., et al. "Effects of the DASH Diet Alone and in Combination with Exercise and Weight Loss on Blood Pressure and Cardiovascular Biomarkers in Men and Women with High Blood Pressure." Archives of Internal Medicine 170:2 (January 25, 2010): 126–135. http://www.ncbi.nlm.nih.gov/pmc/articles/PMC3633078/
16. "Physical Activity Basics." Centers for Disease Control and Prevention. http://www.cdc.gov/physicalactivity/basics/index.htm
17. "4 Types of Exercise." Go4Life from the National Institute on Aging at NIH. https://go4life.nia.nih.gov/4-types-exercise
18. "DASH Diet: Tips for Dining Out." Mayo Clinic. http://www.mayoclinic.org/healthy-lifestyle/nutrition-and-healthy-eating/in-depth/dash-diet/art-20044759
19. "Health Benefits of Smoothies." The Science of Eating. http://thescienceofeating.com/healthy-drinks/benefits-of-smoothies/
20. "Detoxification." Partnership for Environmental Education and Rural Health. http://peer.tamu.edu/curriculum_modules/OrganSystems/Module_3/index.htm

Conversions

TEMPERATURE CONVERSIONS

FAHRENHEIT (°F)	CELSIUS (°C)
325°F	165°C
350°F	175°C
375°F	190°C
400°F	200°C
425°F	220°C
450°F	230°C

VOLUME CONVERSIONS

U.S.	U.S. EQUIVALENT	METRIC
1 tablespoon (3 teaspoons)	½ fluid ounce	15 milliliters
¼ cup	2 fluid ounces	60 milliliters
⅓ cup	3 fluid ounces	90 milliliters
½ cup	4 fluid ounces	120 milliliters
⅔ cup	5 fluid ounces	150 milliliters
¾ cup	6 fluid ounces	180 milliliters
1 cup	8 fluid ounces	240 milliliters
2 cups	16 fluid ounces	480 milliliters

WEIGHT CONVERSIONS

U.S.	METRIC
½ ounce	15 grams
1 ounce	30 grams
2 ounces	60 grams
¼ pound	115 grams
⅓ pound	150 grams
½ pound	225 grams
¾ pound	350 grams
1 pound	450 grams

INDEX

RECIPE INDEX

ABOUT THE AUTHOR

Kate Barrington graduated from Marietta College in 2009 with a Bachelor's Degree in English and a focus in creative writing. Since then she has built a business for herself as a freelance writer specializing in health and fitness niche topics. Kate loves to explore new diets and fitness trends while also putting her passion for food to work in crafting original recipes for cookbooks and diet guides. Kate takes her role as a nonfiction writer very seriously and views every project as an opportunity to learn something new and to share her knowledge with readers around the globe.